620319

"Black Rover, Come Over!"

UNIVERSITY OF ILLINOIS PRESS Urbana Chicago London

"Black Rover, Come Over!"

The Hypnosymbolic Treatment of a Phobia

C. Scott Moss and
Pauline James

Manufactured in the United States of America
Library of Congress Catalog Card No. 76-110421

252 00109 5

Contents

Foreword

As everyone knows, when Freud published *Interpretation of Dreams* (1900), he regarded dreams as being "the royal road to the unconscious." In a later foreword to a revised edition he wrote, "Insight such as this falls to one's lot but once in a lifetime." [1] I believed what Freud said about dreams providing him with entry into psychogenetic factors that were outside of the patient's waking awareness and to the dynamics which underlay the patient's symptoms. Over the past 20 years, I have attempted to perfect the use of hypnosis in dream translation to facilitate psychotherapy.

It seems to me that I have accumulated considerable evidence that a primary value of hypnosis in psychotherapy is that it allows access to the symbol-translating mechanism. For example, recall of a forgotten dream may be enhanced by hypnotic revivification, an interrupted dream may

[1] Sigmund Freud, *The Interpretation of Dreams*, ed. J. Strachey (New York: Basic Books, 1960).

be carried to completion, and some hypnotized subjects will respond to the suggestion "to dream" about their conflict areas, while others display an ability to interpret symbolic material.

While I am particularly concerned about spontaneous night dreams and not "dreams" that are produced in the hypnotic sessions themselves (they seem rather prosiac products), one cannot pretend that even nocturnal dreams are uncontaminated by psychotherapy. Most therapy dreams fall into a special category. They are not as simple and mundane as the usual dreams obtained by investigations in electrophysiological studies. They seem, instead, to provide the patient with an auxiliary form of communication to speak of things that he is not yet ready to commit to conventional language or even to think of in the usual waking manner.

I am eclectic, not psychoanalytic, by orientation; for example, I don't adhere to the psychoanalytic structure of the personality (id-ego-super-ego) nor do I delve at length into the psychoarcheology of the patient's infancy. I also do not emphasize the analysis of transference which is absolutely crucial to psychoanalysis. I deviate from other psychoanalytic concepts as well. Whereas Freud valued dreams as providing access to the infantile sources of conflict and he placed demand upon his patients for a *linear* type of free association leading back to the infantile substructure, the hypnotic therapist employs a *radial* type of association to amplify the immediate meaning of each dream element (à la Jung). In addition, I learned that symbolism is always unique to the individual patient rather than possessing anything akin to universal symbolism. The free association almost always relates to the here-and-now of current problem situations.

Very early I learned that while the therapist is *directive* in structuring the situation in which symbols can be produced (setting the stage with hypnosis), he must become highly *nondirective* in either attempting to produce the content or in the interpretation of the dreams themselves. The production of the dreams and the translation of the symbols must be the patient's responsibility. The therapist becomes relatively directive again in the effort to integrate what the patient says about his dreams back into his conflicted life pattern.

The fundamental point in hypnosymbolic treatment is that in dealing with a person's dreams, you are dealing with content which contains a high degree of emotional imagery. *There is no such thing as a neutral symbol — when you deal with symbols, you are dealing with highly charged affective meaning.* Dealing with dreams under hypnosis brings them alive again and a corrective emotional experience ensues. It is much more than dealing with intellectual insight. Once you know what the symptoms (in this case, the phobia) really mean, then you are in a position to employ what behavior therapists now call reinforcement principles to remedy the underlying pathology.

This report is of the brief, successful treatment of a phobic reaction in which the patient's repressive defenses were penetrated, leading to a simple, convincing demonstration of the childhood learning of the phobic response and its subsequent ramifications. A symbolic fantasy procedure, tailored to the patient's unique personality dynamics, was then instituted in order to consolidate the obtained insights and further desensitize the patient to the fear-provoking stimuli. The actual content of the report was largely written by the patient. She surprised me at the end of therapy by presenting me with a lengthy narrative which reveals the richness of the treatment experience from her viewpoint. (My formal account is contained in the book, *Dreams, Images, and Fantasy: A Semantic Differential Casebook*, 1970.) In addition, a tape has been prepared which attempts to capture the highlights of her psychotherapeutic experience. A transcript of this recording appears on pp. 91–140.

C. Scott Moss

The Patient's Personal Story

PAULINE JAMES

This story began in a brown leather chair in the doctor's office at the Clinic Building of the state mental hospital. Or maybe it didn't. Maybe it began forty years ago with a very small child. I am not sure that I know.

I could never remember a time when I was not afraid of dogs. Not just a vague, mild anxiety, but an acute, shuddering uneasiness. Not a fear of being bitten, but of something unnameable. Not as much afraid of the larger, slower-moving animal as of the smaller, more active puppy. But always afraid. I can remember crossing the street three or four times in one block because a dog did so, and I wanted to be on the side opposite from it.

Not only as a child did I do this, but also as an adult. I can recall turning down many dinner invitations because I knew that the hostess had a house dog, and days of uneasiness before going to a dinner party, wondering if the hostess might have a dog. I remember a night spent with friends. Since the last visit they had acquired a dog. They knew of my fear so they said the dog would sleep in the basement instead of in their little boy's bedroom. I fell asleep easily for I knew that I was on one floor and the dog on another and that a closed door separated us. However, during the night a thunderstorm came up and the frightened little boy wanted his dog. His mother knew that the dog would not harm me and did the only sensible thing from her viewpoint. She did not know that one of her guests did not sleep for the rest of the night. I reacted foolishly and I knew it, but was completely helpless to do otherwise.

As I grew older I realized that this fear was peculiar to me. Other people did not have it. I was normal enough to realize that, in this way at least, I was abnormal. I tried to reason my fear away. I tried to find out why I had always lived in the shadow of this haunting, ever-present fear. I asked my parents if they knew why I was afraid. I could not recall ever having been frightened or hurt by a dog.

My mother felt that she had the explanation and told me of this incident. Just before I was born my brother, who was four years old, was playing under the kitchen table. The family dog, which was kept outside, found the door open and wandered in. My mother discovered him under the table with my brother, immediately realized that the dog had gone mad, and that not only her boy but the rest of the family was in real danger. Acting upon impulse, she got the dog outside the door and called to my father who was working in the field nearby. She was terribly frightened as she kept one eye on the dog and one eye on my father while he crossed to get to a neighbor's house where he could borrow a gun. It appeared, two or three times, as if the dog might attack my father. She told me how she watched from the window while my father shot and killed the family pet, the dog which seemed almost like a member of the family. This, she said, was the cause of my fear.

It seemed a plausible explanation at the time, but my fear persisted in spite of it. It seemed a likely explanation, that is, until I was old enough to read that it had been proved conclusively that a mother's fears cannot be transmitted to her unborn child. So I kept looking for some other explanation. I felt very keenly that if I could recall or find out why I was afraid, I could conquer the fear. But the "why" always evaded me and the terrible fear persisted. One cannot fight the unknown.

In college I took all the psychology and philosophy courses they offered, and I was especially interested in abnormal psychology. Maybe I was hoping that there I could find the solution to this gnawing thing that had more or less dominated my life for as long as I could remember.

The realization came slowly that this fear was something I could not defeat by myself. I think a faint hope was stirred within me when there seemed to emerge a new kind of doctor. The words "psychiatrist" and "psychoanalyst" were being used normally, not with the stigma of the previous years in which these men were regarded as perhaps the descendants of witch-doctors and dealt only with the feeble-minded and those broken pieces of humanity that families wanted to hide away from an inquisitive society. I read everything I could find about what these new doctors were doing. A very general impression that people had of them was that they were a new professional class — a luxury for the idle rich or for the frustrated conversationalist in need of a listener, a rather aloof and somewhat superior individual who had replaced the Magic Carpet with a more luxurious Magic Couch, one who half-listened to imaginary complaints, collected exorbitant fees, and left the patient feeling a little better, the doctor a little richer, and perhaps both a little happier.

Believe me, it does not work that way. In the first place, my doctor had no luxurious couch. In fact, no couch at all. Rather, an old brown leather chair that tended to be more uncomfortable than comfortable. He was not aloof. He exhibited no feelings of superiority. He was certainly not a half-interested listener. And I felt that he was working as hard and with as much dedication to save my emotional life as a surgeon works to save his patient's life in the operating room. To the patient there is very little difference: some abnormal growth or diseased organ is being removed and it makes small difference whether the surgeon or the psychiatrist does it. There is one difference, however. The surgeon has an anesthetic to lessen the pain — the psychiatrist or psychologist has none.

Since the Second World War there has been an ever increasing interest in mental health. The general public was made to realize that a mental illness is no more to be ashamed of than a physical illness. The public also came to realize that there are varying degrees of mental disturbances — just as in physical ailments there is the slight cold and there is cancer. I hoped my phobia would compare to the slight cold class. I do not know whether it did.

All the time I kept wondering: if I wouldn't be able to lose my fear, could I find someone who could help me learn why I was afraid? I had not yet met Dr. M. but my opportunity was finally to come.

We had moved to a small college town which also held one of the state's largest mental institutions. Several psychologists from the hospital taught some of the courses at the college where we taught, so we got to know them. More than once, I had thought of mentioning my dog phobia to one of them but the opportunity didn't seem to come. One night, however, we were seated in the local theater watching *The Three Faces of Eve*, when Dr. W. came in and sat down beside us. After the show, it was quite natural to fall into a discussion of the movie. I recall Dr. W.'s saying that perhaps we see people every day who have some tendencies similar to those of Eve, and that most of us had our own little quirks of one kind or another. Here was the chance I had waited for. It was easy to tell him about my fear and to ask him if he thought anyone could help me understand why I was afraid. I think I suggested that maybe hypnosis could do it and asked if any of the doctors at the hospital were interested in it. I had read as much as a lay person can about hypnosis and I really believed the incident, if there was one, lay buried in my subconscious. For I had probed into my conscious memories and could find nothing to account for the fear, but the fear remained. I rather expected that way down beyond the point of recall was some episode where my older brothers had perhaps gleefully, and for fun, caused their dog to chase and frighten me. I was totally unprepared for what was really buried there.

Dr. W. seemed interested in my case and said he would take it up with another doctor who just might be able to help me. On Saturday I thought about the conversation with Dr. W. once or twice, then forgot it. On Sunday he called to say that the head of the Psychology Service was interested in my problem, that hypnosis was an interest of his, and that he would be happy to see me if I cared to make an appointment.

Session I, Thursday, January 23

I was a bit nervous about my first trip to the state hospital. I had not been inside any of the buildings except an auditorium where we had heard Dr. Milton Erickson speak on medical hypnosis. In fact, it was at this lecture that I had become more keenly interested in learning whether hypnosis could dig down through the rubble of my subconscious and find the key to my problem. If Dr. Erickson had called for a volunteer that night I would have gone up to the platform, that is how interested I was. I guess I thought he could uncover my problem in a five- or ten-minute session. Apparently my husband sensed my uneasiness about this first visit and offered to accompany me. I was greatly relieved.

If I had expected to meet some obvious mental cases in the halls, I was to be surprised. To this day I'm not positive, in many instances, who are the employees and who are the patients. Of course, I am sure that there are buildings where the difference is more obvious. Or maybe not. Not long ago I heard the famed psychoanalyst and Freud's biographer, Dr. Ernest Jones, say on TV that he had yet to meet a completely normal person: that in a sense the abnormal was really the normal. And Karl and William Menninger have both written and said that the line separating the mentally ill and the mentally healthy is very fine, indeed.

When we went into Dr. M.'s office we had a few minutes to wait before he came in. It looked like any other office. A large desk piled high with work yet to be done. I have since learned that he is a very busy man. There was a straight chair, a wash basin in one corner, drapes at the window, a piece of pottery that perhaps some patient had made in occupational therapy, and of course, the big brown leather chair. There was a small metal box on the desk which interested us. We decided that it was probably some sort of intercom system. I secretly wondered if it might be there so he could call a guard if a patient got out of control. Little did I guess that that little microphone would record on tape every word that I said during my sessions for the next several weeks while I sat in the brown leather chair and relived my life.

While we waited we heard music coming from down the hall. Someone was playing the piano, someone a drum, and there were other instruments. The music was not too bad, perhaps a bit loud. Occasionally an interesting voice would join in. It sounded as if it had at one time been trained. Some tones had good full quality — others were extremely strained. The music was all jazz and when the voice plaintively sang "The Birth of the Blues," there seemed to be pathos and heartbreak — real — not just assumed as blues singers are so apt to do. And we wondered. When the doctor came he told us that this was music therapy. I have often wondered about the voice. I wonder about the person and the sadness in her voice. I wonder just what had put it there. Is she, too, reliving her life trying to find out what has caused the hurt?

I was a bit surprised when I met Dr. M. Maybe I had expected someone with a goatee and piercing black eyes, for isn't that the way a hypnotist should look? He looked just like any young man you might meet anywhere. I had expected an older man.

I told him as much as I could about my problem: simply that I was afraid of dogs and had been for as long as there was any memory. He said he would try to help me, but that he couldn't promise. He asked me what I thought of hypnosis and remarked that not everyone was a good hypnotic subject. I asked him what the determining factors were and if he thought I would be a good subject. He said we would try to find out that afternoon. He asked if I were certain that this was something I really wanted to do.

I assured him that I had wanted to find help for a long time, but more than ever now. I explained that we had a young daughter who wanted a puppy very badly and I wanted her to have one — except for the awful fear. I thought that perhaps an only child is apt to be lonely and that the puppy, which she wanted, would dispel her loneliness. (In the weeks that were to follow I was to learn that even a small child in a large family, with a puppy of her own, can also be very lonely.)

Dr. M. asked if I would take a test or two. I was to look at pictures and make up a story about each of them. I recalled an evening several years ago when a friend of ours, who was completing his doctorate in psychology, had brought his set of Rorschach cards to the house and we had all looked at the colorful blots. I remembered that we were all somewhat reluctant to say just what the pictures made us think of lest we discover undesirable tendencies that we didn't know we had. I recalled the friend's saying that it was always safe to call the blots flowers or butterflies or something — but for the life of me I couldn't recall the safe answer. I was relieved when Dr. M.'s test was not the Rorschach test. His consisted of some rather interesting studies of animals, mostly dogs, I believe. One or two of them had rather good art quality and I became interested in that phase of them too.

Another test consisted of mimeograph sheets listing various groups of opposites, such as plain or striking, happy or sad, weak or strong, hard or soft, etc. I was to check these as they pertained to my feelings about cats, dogs, father, mother, self, and the doctor. I kept getting mixed up as to whether I was checking my feelings or my objective ideas about them.

Dr. M. said we would then try to find out whether I was a good hypnotic subject. He told me to get comfortable in the brown leather chair, to close my eyes and to try to relax. He explained that hypnosis was sort of like the stage between being wide awake and deeply asleep. That surprised me for I had thought that, under hypnosis, one was deeply asleep and completely oblivious to his surroundings. He said I would be aware of things going on around me but that I was not to pay attention to them. Rather, he said, I should concentrate on his voice. He did not tell me to stare into his eyes. Neither did he swing a watch back and forth in front of my face. He just told me to close my eyes and relax. It seems he told me that we were going down a thickly carpeted stairway — slowly — one step at a time. Then there was something about my being in a canoe on a lazy summer's day — just drifting downstream. I felt as if I really were. And I recalled a summer many years ago when a group of us canoed regularly on the lakes at Forest Park in St. Louis. I was becoming very relaxed and sleepy. I seemed to feel the warmth of the summer's sun as it shone down upon me as I lazily drifted farther and farther downstream. It seemed especially welcome, I guess, for this first visit with Dr. M. took place in the dead of winter. I heard a phone ring in the outer office but it did not disturb me. I recall Dr. M.'s saying that in order to save time during future visits he would give me some suggestions to cause a deep hypnosis to be arrived at more quickly. I recall his saying that each time he would rap on his desk with a pencil I would feel an overpowering urge to fall deeper asleep. (This was to cause a humorous and somewhat embarrassing situation before long.)

A couple of incidents during this initial experience especially interested me. At one phase the doctor told me that my eyelids had become so heavy that it would be impossible for me to open my eyes. I tried to, but it was as if they were glued down tightly. At another point, he said my fingers were so tightly locked together that it would be impossible to pull them apart. He was so right, for I tried that too. Yet I felt that I could if I had really wanted to.

Dr. M. told me, just before he awakened me, that he would recite the alphabet to the letter "E," and I would awaken gradually and be wide awake and feeling fine when he reached "E." It worked just that way too. I awakened, felt fine and a little surprised, I guess, that I had actually experienced hypnosis. I remember feeling relieved that I had apparently passed the first test for being an acceptable subject. I had new hope now that maybe I could lose my fear of dogs.

Just as we were leaving [the session] I mentioned something that had bothered me for several years. About ten years ago I had heard something in a delivery room that I had very much wanted to remember. I recalled, down through the years, that it had seemed very important at the time that I remember it. However, the intervening years had dulled the compulsion to remember and now it only bothered me occasionally. I asked Dr. M. if, since we were going back some forty years to my earliest childhood of which I had no recollection, we could make a stop ten years back and try to recapture this lost memory.

During the next few days I thought a great deal about this forgotten something. The feeling that I had experienced during the weeks immediately following the delivery room incident seemed to come back. However, the events of about two years or more seemed to merge and only the need to remember stood out as clearly as it had ten years ago. I could recall quite vividly that while I was in the delivery room I heard something that no one thought I had — and they didn't think I would ever repeat it. I knew at the time they were wrong — that I must remember it so I could tell my husband. I could remember an almost happy feeling at being able to outwit them. But once back in my hospital room, I realized that the thing I wanted so badly to remember was gone. I could not recall it. For weeks, I would lie awake at night reconstructing the whole situation, hoping, I guess, to sneak up on the remark that eluded me. Sometimes I just about had it, but always it would move out of grasp. I recalled that one time, shortly after the incident, I had asked the head nurse of the OB section what it was that I had heard and could not recall. I felt that she would know, for she had stayed with me through the long and difficult delivery. She had become a close friend of mine and I thought she could tell me, but she only looked at me for a moment or two and said, "Don't try any longer to recall it — it's better not to."

I didn't give up that easily. But the passing years took care of it and the need to remember seemed diminished, though it never went away entirely.

I looked forward to the next meeting with Dr. M. I guess I thought he could just pull an isolated incident from my subconscious, like a rabbit out of a hat, but I was to learn how very wrong this idea was. I was to learn that forgetting is one of the kindest blessings of mankind. The days before my next visit were rather uneventful and before I knew it Monday had arrived.

Therapist's Summary of Session I

The patient, aged 45, an art instructor, appeared in company with her husband. She stated that she had recently seen the movie, *The Three Faces of Eve*, and it finally had encouraged her to seek treatment for a lifelong, intense fear of dogs. She was also motivated by the desire to present her daughter with a puppy on the occasion of her ninth birthday, two weeks hence. She requested that, as in the movie, hypnosis be used to uncover the source of her phobia.

The patient made a generally favorable initial prognostic impression, seeming to be an intelligent, well-educated, sensitive person. The problem seemed relatively circumscribed and her current environmental adjustment was adequate. I was slightly disconcerted by the husband's presence. She explained that the reason she had brought him was because she feared that under hypnosis she might say something that the therapist would not tell her. I could have asked him to wait outside before beginning the hypnotic induction, but since the wife was anxious that he remain, I asked him instead to participate in the session. He subsequently listened to my instructions to his wife but didn't become hypnotized himself.

Her response to initial induction procedures was favorable, and I agreed that treatment would be undertaken for a maximum of seven to eight sessions over a three-week period. The remainder of the session was spent in training her in rapid entry into hypnosis. At the conclusion of the hour, she asked that the attempt be made first to recapture the lost memory of "something important" that had occurred during the birth of a child ten years ago. Although I had no idea what she was looking for (and she couldn't tell me), I did have confidence that it related to her phobia and so I readily accepted her suggestion.

Session II, Monday, January 27

This was the beginning of term examinations at the college and my husband was unusually busy. He had a conference he couldn't postpone so he was unable to accompany me to my appointment with Dr. M. I was disappointed and even thought of changing my appointment. Later I was glad I had not done so.

This time it seemed easier to slip into hypnosis. The raps on the desk with a pencil made me feel very sleepy. I seem to recall now that there were more carpeted stairs to go down and finally an elevator descent. I can recall a feeling of curiosity about what would be down there. It seemed that there was a dark hallway with lots of doors on either side, and although the doors were identical, the one just to the left of where I stood seemed to hold a peculiar interest for me. We opened it and went in. I say "we," for I didn't feel alone. It seemed as if Dr. M. was there beside me.

The inside of the room was dark, but there was a window which revealed sunshine outside. Both in the hall and in this room there seemed to be light only at the exact spot where I stood. Through the window I could see a blue sky, a green countryside, and bright sunshine. It seemed to be June. As I looked around inside the room which had first appeared to be empty, it took on more meaning. The darkness was replaced by bright light. A hospital cart stood in one corner. This was a delivery room, the delivery room where I might find, at last, the words that had kept eluding me for ten years. This was the stop ten years back that I had wanted to make.

But the years have a way of running together, much the way water paints blend on a wet surface, and I didn't know whether this was the delivery room of ten or eleven years ago. I had been there, in the same room, both times in June, and I wasn't even sure anymore which time it was that I had heard the phrase I had wanted so badly to recall.

Under hypnosis these two years became disentangled and started to come into clear focus, as when one adjusts a pair of binoculars. I was again experiencing the delivery room scene, or scenes. For I had to relive both of them before I could find what I had been looking for. The first incident was a happy one. My little daughter had been delivered rather easily and I felt a joy and a sense of achievement that caused me to be happier than I had ever been before.

Recalling this happy experience brought with it many forgotten incidents. I could see the beautiful summer day that was to be my baby's birthday. I had awakened as usual but soon discovered symptoms that caused me to call the doctor. He had me come to his office, saw me before the other waiting patients. This worried me a little, for in a small town you know everybody and I hated going ahead of these people. I recalled that his wife, a friend of mine, was helping him that morning for his regular nurse was ill. I remembered her telling me of their meeting in the hospital out East where she trained and he interned. The doctor sent me directly to the hospital in the city about ten miles away. We went by way of the old road, instead of the new four-lane highway. I always enjoyed the pastoral scenes which we viewed from the old road. We picked up one of the students who was hitchhiking to the city. It was a beautiful day. I was not too uncomfortable, and it was to be the birthday of our child. I recalled thinking how surprised the student would be if he knew the purpose of our trip into town. I was very, very happy.

The day progressed without much excitement and I was afraid the doctor would send me home. I felt sort of put out because they wouldn't give me lunch. I had been hungry for the past few months, so hungry, in fact, that I had told my husband not to bring me flowers when I went to the hospital, but rather something to eat. He did too. Next morning he baked a beautiful cake and decorated it with my name and the name we had chosen if our baby should be a girl. But the excitement of motherhood had done away with my hunger and I completely lost my appetite. The nurses enjoyed the cake. I recalled that after the delivery that evening, the doctor and my husband left for a late dinner at one of the city's nicer restaurants, and told me to sleep. But I was too happy and excited to sleep.

Many things I recalled — the tarnished happiness a few days later at learning that I was to go home on Wednesday, but that my little daughter would have to remain in the hospital a few days longer. I didn't want to go home and leave her. The pediatrician explained that since she was so tiny they would like to keep her awhile. I rather resented this since my doctor had practically starved me in order to produce a small baby. Perhaps there was more fear than resentment, however, for I sensed that all was not well.

I recalled that late Friday afternoon — just one week after our baby's birth — the doctor stopped by the house and asked for my husband. I told him he was at the hospital visiting our baby. He said he would see him there. His manner seemed strained and strange. I was worried.

I recalled that about two hours later my neighbor said my husband had phoned to say the baby seemed better. In less than a half hour, however, she came back to tell me that our baby had died. I couldn't believe it. For there in the corner was the crib waiting for her, and beside it was the chest containing all of her clothes. I resented my neighbor's telling me. I felt she should have waited for my husband to do it. Maybe I thought it might hurt less that way. I know now that it would have made little difference who told me. It was a cruel fact that could not be changed.

The minister came and said he knew exactly how we felt, for he had nearly lost his child. I told him that he did not know how we felt, for he had only nearly lost his child. We *had* lost ours. My heart had its share of bitterness, but from the minister's remark I learned a valuable lesson: that we cannot truly sympathize with another or understand his sorrow unless we have experienced an identical sorrow or trouble ourselves. Perhaps the Indians knew this when they said, "Don't judge another's actions unless you have walked in his moccasins for a day."

I recalled our taking our baby to St. Louis to bury it beside the son we had lost four years earlier. I recalled the doctor's saying I must not make the trip, and his coming back the next morning to say his wife had convinced him it would be better for me to go than to remain behind alone.

I recalled the many friends who went with us to the station in Jackson and that I was weary as we waited for the train. I recalled looking down at the bright lights of Main Street (for the station is above street level) and my husband's saying, "You don't think you will ever smile again, but you will." I didn't understand how he could even think of smiling. I know now that he understood more about time's healing process than I did. I recalled that just before the train came a baggage cart passed nearby and everyone tried to divert my attention. But I saw the tiny box that contained the body of our baby anyhow. I thought of how we had planned to take our baby home and proudly show it to our relatives and friends. It was not like this.

I recalled that the train came and that the football coach carried me from the wheel chair to the berth that had already been made up; that the coach who had been like a brother to both of us reached down, kissed me on the cheek, and said in his slow Southern accent, "Keep yo chin up, heah? We'll be sayin' a prayer for you." There was a tear in the eye of the coach who the boys thought was so tough.

I remembered the welcome coolness of the air-conditioned train, for June in Mississippi is very warm. I remembered sleeping fitfully. The sedative that the doctor gave was too mild. The train stopped at Carbondale where some cars would be taken off for the Chicago part of the trip. My husband went outside to make sure the baby's body was left on the right section of the train. I was uneasy lest he not get back on the train before it started. I raised the shade and looked out into the night. I could see the hospital about a half block away where my older sister had died a few years ago. I felt as if there had never been and never would be any happiness in my life.

I recalled so many things. I was also learning that one cannot recapture an isolated incident from one's past; that all is so interwoven; that many things must be remembered if one wants to find a particular incident; that not even hypnosis can brush aside all but one specific incident. Remembering is a more complicated process.

I recalled being at the cemetery burying the baby. A college classmate, now a prominent minister, was speaking. Instead of paying attention to him I was remembering a day about four years earlier. We had buried our first child then and I had come back to visit the grave before joining my soldier-husband who had to return to Fort Sam Houston after a very short leave. As I stood there feeling sorry for myself I noticed a plot nearby that contained the graves of two babies. I thought, and maybe said aloud, "I can stand having one tiny grave here, but that I just could not stand: I couldn't stand having two." We are fortunate that the future is withheld from us.

I dreaded returning to our home in Mississippi. It would seem so empty compared to the happiness we had expected with our little girl. But after the two weeks that the president of the college had given my husband, it was time for him to resume his teaching. Although it must have been difficult for him to have much enthusiasm for his work now, I rather envied him his classes. He could get away from the empty house. I seemed to be a prisoner in it.

The neighbor whom I had resented because she told me of my baby's death had rearranged our house the way it was before we had made plans for the baby. All the things that would remind us had been carefully put away. We appreciated this and I was ashamed of my earlier resentment.

Life must go on and we tried to get interested in things. We swam, played some golf and tennis, but nothing was much fun anymore. We made fig preserves and took care of the botany professor's hydroponic garden while he was away. It was interesting, I guess, but not much fun. Friends urged me to have some children's art classes. I did.

I recalled that the president asked me to teach an art class at the college. I hesitated for I thought he asked me just because he felt sorry for me. Finally, however, I said I would and started making plans for a course that was new to the curriculum. There was considerable interest in the course and art has been taught there ever since. I remembered one likable young man who wanted to become an interior decorator, but who had a yellow complex and did every project predominantly yellow.

I had an interest now, and a job to do. Things were a little better. Also, we had contacted the Mississippi Children's Home and had begun steps toward adoption. We had gotten together all the necessary data, had been visited in our home, which was modest but seemed acceptable to the social worker. We were warned that the waiting period was at least two years. That seemed a long way off, but it was something to hope for.

Then I recalled a day in early September. As we were coming out of the building where we had our classes, we were met by a young student whom we had not seen since the close of school in late May. I felt again the horrible feeling that engulfed me as she asked, "How is that little baby of yours?" I recalled her embarrassment as my husband calmly explained what had happened.

I was also learning in the process of remembering that we not only forget the unhappiness in our lives but the more pleasant things as well. I was remembering the many friends who did so much to try to help us find our way out of the valley of disappointment.

All of these memories that had been so deftly hidden away were bared for me to see. I had wanted it so. I had wanted so badly to find one misplaced phrase. Now I wasn't sure that it was worth it. I was struggling with myself. I wanted to find the lost phrase, but I wasn't sure that I wanted to pay the necessary price of reliving so many unhappy incidents. I decided to steel myself against the hurt and search on. But "what fools we mortals be." It was not possible to relive the old memories without also experiencing the old hurt. I could not steel myself against it.

[Under hypnosis] I went back into the room on the left, this time to relive the events of the delivery of June of the next year. Apparently it was there that the secret of the forgotten words was hidden. I remember now that Dr. M. asked if I still wanted to go through with this and I said I did. The incidents concerning this later trip to the delivery room were coming into clearer focus. I could see the doctor plainly and remember his name. I had tried unsuccessfully to recall it a few weeks earlier.

That day in June started like any other. I had been X-rayed the day before and told to return in two weeks. We had stopped in the city for dinner and a movie and had stayed up late talking to friends. I had not been awake long when I knew we had to call the doctor. He sent an ambulance immediately and the sirens screamed all the way into the city. They need not have hurried. There were to be long hours of waiting.

As the day wore on I knew that things were not going well. The doctor, a very fine specialist, stayed with me all day. I remembered being concerned because he did not go out to eat. Once he said he was going out into the hall to see my husband and report what was happening. After a while the nurse listened for the baby's heartbeat with a stethoscope, looked concerned, and called the doctor. I suggested that he do a Caesarean. He said it was too late. He told the anesthetist to tell him when she was ready. Then, under hypnosis, I heard something that I didn't ever remember hearing before. It confused me. The doctor said, "If we wait, she may go too." I could not understand that. Although it was a long and abnormal delivery, I was never at any time aware of any actual danger to myself. I was aware of danger to the baby, however. This seemed to be the phrase I had not been able to recall. At least it was something I had never remembered hearing. I was disappointed for it didn't seem that important. The compulsion to remember seemed all out of proportion to the thing remembered. Many things kept coming back, clear and in their proper order and I was glad to leave this room on the left side of the dark hallway. I was glad to hear Dr. M. say, "In a few minutes I will awaken you. Sleep deeply and awaken feeling rested." On the letter "E" I was wide awake, but I had a feeling of sadness that I had not taken with me into hypnosis. It was something that had followed me as I returned from the dark hallway of many doors. I awakened thinking about the doctor who had been caring for me during my first pregnancy. His name had also been Dr. M. We had always wondered if that venture might have ended more happily had it been possible to stay under his care. But those were war years and everybody's lives and plans were being altered. I remembered how hard we had worked in order that my husband could complete a Ph.D. degree before his draft notice came; how happy we had been about the pregnancy; how he had turned down a commission in the Navy in order to have the two months needed to complete his thesis; how we treasured those two months together. I remembered the conferring of the degree, but that the happiness of the occasion was dimmed by the conferring of a private's rank in the Army just two days before. I had not thought about any of this for a very long time.

I recall now that Dr. M. asked me how I felt and I replied that I felt all right but depressed. He said it was probably because of the content of the material we had covered. I agreed. We made an appointment for the next Friday. I left the brown leather chair much sadder than when I sat down in it. I was glad my husband had not come along. He, too, would have been saddened by this session.

The sadness that I carried with me [after session II] was so real that I lost my appetite and I couldn't sleep. This is the way I have always reacted to the deep emotional experiences of my life. I was not only recalling half-forgotten incidents, as all of us do sometimes, it seemed as if I were actually reliving them! Many times during the next few days I was very close to tears and I do not cry easily. I felt so depressed that I actually felt ill and once the college nurse gave me something for the nausea I felt. I thought about this last visit to the state hospital almost constantly. The depression never completely left me for a minute. The phrase I had heard continued to puzzle me. It just didn't seem important enough to have insisted so strongly upon being remembered.

Finally I talked to my husband about it. We both knew it had been a difficult delivery, but I didn't know until now that he had blamed himself all these years for having discouraged the surgeon's doing a Caesarean section. The college nurse had been a close friend for many years and had served at the college where we were ten years ago. Since she knew something of those years I was reliving, I felt I could talk to her. She explained that very often there is danger in a delivery room which comes quickly and leaves quickly, and that was perhaps what the doctor had observed. Especially since the delivery had been long and hard, there had perhaps been signs of danger, she said. She explained that nurses are taught to expect anything in the delivery room, to be always on guard, and to be ready for any emergency. The remembered phrase seemed to make more sense after talking to her, but it still did not seem important enough to have caused me so much worry.

I told her of my husband's blaming himself about the Caesarean section. She said he had perhaps unwittingly saved my life for there existed, at the time, a pernicious anemia condition which was undiagnosed, thus untreated. She said it was likely that neither child nor mother would have survived the operation because of the low hemoglobin count which the ailment caused. I wonder if this blame which my husband carried was responsible for our watching a surgeon-friend perform a Caesarean section some years later.

Although these days were darkened with depression there was one humorous incident that occurred. On Thursday, my craft class had gotten to the stage of their leather work where they used stamping tools. A design is impressed upon the dampened leather by striking the tool with a wooden mallet. It sounded exactly as when Dr. M. would rap on his desk with a pencil in order to hasten the hypnosis process. I became sleepier with each mallet stroke until I could stand it no longer. I dismissed my class early, thinking that once outside in the fresh air, I would be all right. I yawned every few seconds as I walked across the campus toward home and continued yawning as often after I got home. I wanted very badly to go to sleep but couldn't for there remained only a couple of hours before we had to attend a formal dinner, and I had yet to help our little girl with her music and her homework and prepare something for her to eat. I continued to yawn while I did these things.

I got out my prettiest formal and yawned all the while I was dressing. My little girl, who likes to watch me dress for parties, commented that I surely did look sleepy. We got to the dinner and I continued to yawn. I could not help myself. The hostess was concerned and I think my husband was somewhat ashamed of me. The hostess asked the waitress to bring coffee with my meal, but at our formal college dinners coffee is not served until dessert and the waitress was reluctant to violate the rule. This embarrassed the hostess, but I assured her I understood. I had waited tables while in college so I knew how the student felt about violating the rules. I just continued to yawn. I was glad that we have only candle light at the formal dinners. At least only the people at our table were aware of my predicament. With dessert came the coffee, but it did not help any. I continued to yawn. We went over to the auditorium where I yawned and half slept through one of the best recitals of the year. Sidney Harth, noted American violinist who recently placed second in the International Music Festival, was the guest artist. And I could not stay awake and hear him.

During the reception that followed I did little or no better. I just wanted to get home, into bed, and go to sleep. When I got there, however, I could not go to sleep. There seemed to be segments of my life that I had yet to remember before my visit with Dr. M. the next day, so I stayed awake most of the night remembering.

Next day I wanted to verify some of the memories that had seemed vague. Fortunately I had the family diary that my husband has always so carefully kept. Although there were many recordings of my discouragement, there were some other things I should have read long ago. Attached to the page bearing the date of our wedding anniversary were two lovely poems, clipped and put there, no doubt, so that I might find them and derive some needed comfort and assurance of love and understanding. I did not need the poems to tell me that; however, I am sorry I had to wait ten years to find them. Each of us was trying to hide our grief from the other. Each of us refrained from mentioning the loss of our babies knowing it caused the other pain, so for the first time a wall had appeared between us. Not a high wall, for we could reach over it, but a barrier, nevertheless. And each of us felt alone. Grief is a very personal experience and each must find his way through it alone, but here were these poems put there to make it a bit easier for me. They had waited ten years for me to find them.

Among the forgotten fragments of memory was something about a hospital ward with several beds and it seemed to relate to the delivery room episode. It was a vague but worrisome memory. It wouldn't quite come clear and it wouldn't go away. My husband couldn't recall anything about a hospital room with several beds either. Both times I had had private rooms. The memory kept nagging until I again got out the family diary and found the year and months pertaining to the incident we had been investigating. Finally I found it. On the date January 10, was this entry: "Pauline rushed by ambulance to hospital. Threatened miscarriage. Very nauseated and in pain." Then I could recall it all clearly. I had been given the choice of a private room or a ward with several other people. There had been considerable difference in cost so I had chosen the latter. I could recall the doctor's obvious displeasure when he saw what I had taken. It proved a wise choice, however, for the other patients would call a nurse when I was too ill to do so.

I had mixed feelings about returning to the brown leather chair. I half dreaded my appointment for that afternoon and yet was anxious to get on with the real reason I had gone to Dr. M. in the first place.

My husband who is usually very considerate was even more so during these past few days. So much so, that I suspected Dr. M. had contacted him. But I guess he just sensed my sadness. When two people have been very close for a long time it is not easy to hide one's feelings. He asked if I wanted him to go with me to this appointment. He seemed a bit surprised when I told him no. Since the last session had been so depressing, I didn't know what to expect from this one and didn't want him to be affected by it. So I went alone.

Therapist's Summary of Session II

At the beginning of the second session in which she came alone (and also for all subsequent sessions), additional training was instituted to insure her cooperation with hypnotic procedures. Following her wish, she was regressed to the delivery scene in 1948. It was revealed that her baby had died during delivery (as had two earlier children), and she believed that she had forgotten some vital fact concerning its death.

However, while she recalled many long-forgotten details, she was unable to recapture the specific memory, though she narrowed it down to something the physician told the nurse immediately following delivery. It was interesting that during the delivery scene, she spontaneously acted *as if* she were again under a general anesthetic. The following posthypnotic suggestion was given: the sought-after memory would gradually enter awareness and if she sincerely wanted to remember it, she could probably do so at the next session.

(No one gets well in the therapy hour — sessions can have only a *catalytic* effect. You see a patient only an hour or two out of the 168 hours in a week. In hypnosymbolic treatment you always leave the patient with a specific problem to focus on or, in the patient's vernacular, a "homework assignment." The patient must take continuing responsibility for working on his problems. The therapist, in turn, must continually judge how much anxiety the patient can experience in working through her various problems.)

Session III, Friday, January 31

I was a bit surprised when Dr. M. suggested that we had better take another look into the delivery room incident. Just in case, he said, that there might have been something we had missed. So down the carpeted stairs — not slowly anymore, but like one running, and to the elevator we went. Then on down to the darkened hallway. Again we opened the door on the left and went in. The same doctor, the same nurses, and the same hospital cart were there. And, of course, the same patient. Many things that I had not yet recalled about this experience began to come into clear focus. I heard a baby crying in the delivery room and asked if it were a boy or a girl. I thought the delivery was finally over. I was disappointed when the doctor said it was not my baby but one that had been born in an adjoining room and brought into this room for attention since the better equipment was here. I recalled how very quiet it had been in this room when I realized that my baby had been born. The deathly stillness! There should have been a baby's crying! Then I heard the doctor telling the pediatrician to put adrenalin directly into the baby's heart and I knew the reason for the awful stillness. These long-forgotten memories were coming back to me. The next thing I was to hear apparently came from my subconscious. It must have been the phrase that had clamored so long for recognition. This was what I had wanted so desperately to remember. I heard the doctor say very clearly, "Its neck is broken."

There was a feeling of hopelessness and defeat that I had not before experienced. I had known sorrow and discouragement before, but this was more intense. Our hopes for a family had been dashed three times now, and for no apparent reason. Each case had been different. I wondered why the hand that rules our destinies was playing such havoc with our lives. To add to my disappointment I had heard the doctor tell the nurses that I ought not try again because this experience had been too difficult. Previously, I had at least had hope that a future venture might be more successful.

Most of all I dreaded telling my husband that our little boy had not survived. I knew how much this baby meant to him too. We both liked children and had planned a long time ago what we thought to be an ideal family: two boys and two girls. We had now lost two boys and one girl. I recalled my bitterness and wishing I had died too, but recognized it to be a cowardly thought. I remembered being back in my hospital room and the nurse bringing our baby in for us to see. It was wrapped in a blanket and to the casual observer looked like any of the other babies that were carried from the nursery to the mothers' rooms. But there was the all-important difference. Those babies were alive; ours was not. Our baby was perfectly formed and it was hard to believe it was not just asleep. Why had our baby been denied life that had been given to the other babies? My heart was filled with unanswerable questions.

I recalled seeing friends outside my door later that night and wondering why none came in. I recalled that next day my hands were so swollen that I was unable to grasp anything, and that two friends, one younger and one older, stayed with me. They kept bathing my face with cool water, for it was very warm in the room, but I recalled wishing they would go away and leave me alone. I appreciated their kindnesses but I just wanted to be left alone. I thought that once alone, I might be able to find the answer to some of the unanswerable "whys" that were filling my thoughts. I had yet to realize that the same questions that were bothering me have plagued mankind through all the ages. I was yet to realize that what man cannot understand he must learn to accept. I was yet to learn that how we react is more important than what happens to us. I had so much to learn.

I remembered that on the second day a student nurse got mixed up and brought someone's baby into my room. This was the greatest hurt I had received.

Finally Dr. M. awakened me. I felt all right but the same feeling of sadness that had been my constant companion for the last week was still with me. All these hurts that time had so deeply covered I had voluntarily dug up. In spite of the sadness I felt, I knew it had been worth it. I had finally captured the elusive phrase and it was powerless to haunt me any more. I wondered why my nurse friend hadn't told me what it was when I had asked her ten years ago. I knew that the baby had died, and knowing how it died couldn't have hurt too much more. But maybe she thought it would. Or maybe professional ethics had prevented her telling me. Anyhow, I had finally found out.

As I sat in the brown leather chair after Dr. M. awakened me, I felt rather foolish to have considered my dog problem very important after the experience I had just been reliving. Everything else seemed insignificant and trivial but the fact still remained — the fear of dogs was there and I was helpless to do anything about it.

I think I went into hypnosis again during this visit, but I am not sure. It seemed much easier to do each time. I hoped I was becoming an apt pupil. I think Dr. M. told me to keep a pencil and note pad by my bed and to record any dreams I might have before returning for my next session. Even as I was leaving his office some of the depression of the past several days was leaving and some of the old memories seemed content to rest.

The next day was Saturday and a pleasant day. I was beginning to feel more like a normal, happy person again. But I was still remembering. The memories were less directly related to the delivery room incident and more pleasant. I recalled some of the things we did together that summer and fall as we tried to forget our disappointment. I remembered a trip to New Orleans, dinner at Antoinne's, a trip to the Gulf Coast, the beaches at Biloxi and Gulfport. I remembered our Christmas trip to Chicago in our new Oldsmobile, a terrific extravagance! I remembered how much we enjoyed dining in the Empire Room of the Palmer House and our pleasure at listening to the fine string ensemble in person. We had regularly listened to their radio broadcast. I remembered that the menu fascinated us and that we pored over it to find something we could (nearly) afford. I remembered that I was especially interested in the ice-sculptured creations that were displayed on the large table just inside the door, and the most fabulous display of unusual foods we had ever seen. I remembered that we were interested in the portable bars that smart-looking bartenders pulled up to your table to mix your specified drinks. I was a little sorry that neither of us knew enough about mixed drinks to avail ourselves of this privilege.

I remembered our leaving Chicago just as the outer Shore Drive was being closed because the high waves were washing across it. I remembered the excitement of it and that before many miles we had gotten into a blinding snowstorm. Many cars were off the road and a highway officer advised us to turn in at the next town. But the next town had no hotel or motel and the restaurant owner rented us his spare bedroom. I could not go to sleep because I always slept with the window open. My husband obliged by opening it for me and I fell asleep immediately. Next morning we realized that my fresh air fancy had been pretty much imaginary. The inside window was open all right, but a storm window made the room air-tight. We laughed about it.

I remembered things we did with friends: a trip to historic Vicksburg and dinner at the Old Southern Tea Room; a trip to Allison's Wells, a summer resort and artists' colony; spending a night in an old antebellum home (turned guest inn) in Natchez. We took this trip with the coach and his wife and stopped there because of her interest in antiques. One of the two rooms assigned to us contained a bed that Andrew Jackson was supposed to have slept in. The coach's wife was interested in that room because the furniture was older but she felt she should give us the room because of my husband's interest in historical data. We laughed at another possible arrangement for neither the coach nor I had any interests in that room. I remembered a trip to Mobile with the same couple to see the azalea gardens.

And I remembered the things that each of us did separately to try to forget the events of June. My husband decided to take advantage of his GI educational benefits by studying voice and organ. He had always been interested in music and had had a little training in it. He seemed to derive a lot of pleasure from these studies. Every now and then, even yet, I find myself humming a catchy little melody that he wrote while studying organ.

I remembered that while my husband had studied voice and organ my interest returned to piano and painting. I remembered how proud and pleased I had been when he bought a brand new spinet for me.

I remembered the first weekend in March. We had spent it with a student friend and his family. He was a young minister and had asked my husband to speak to his congregation on Sunday. My husband had constantly resisted friends' urgings to become a licensed or ordained minister even though his original reason for going to college was to become a minister. He is a lay speaker and felt early in his college career that he was planning to be a minister simply because everyone expected it, but that his main interest was elsewhere.

We got home late Monday afternoon to learn that the Mississippi Children's Home had been trying to get in touch with us. We had nearly given up hope that they would ever have a child for us and didn't dare to think that this might really be it. We lost no time contacting them. We could scarcely believe it when they said they thought they had the right baby for us, and that we could see her tomorrow and decide. "Her!" We had not specified a preference on our data sheet. This seemed to be the rest of the ideal family we had planned years ago. We spent most of the night getting ready for our little girl. There were many things that had been put away two or three times and now we were finally going to use them. After we had things in order we drove into Jackson and parked outside the Home. It was quite late. We just sat in the car happy that our little girl was inside that house. A light came on in an upstairs window and we wondered if maybe someone were feeding her. And we wondered what she would be like. I remembered our excitement and happiness and how we just did not think we could wait for tomorrow to come.

I recalled that we arrived at the Home a little earlier than the appointed time and were taken into a large parlor. After a few minutes the social worker went upstairs and returned with a tiny pink bundle in her arms. She handed it to me. I had wondered if I would feel the same way about an adopted baby as I would about one born to us. I knew now. I felt exactly as I had when I had held our own little girl in my arms two years before. This was *our baby* too. There was no doubt then, nor has there ever been. I remembered I was surprised to discover that she was so pretty. I'd not thought whether she would be pretty, but here in my arms was the prettiest little baby I had ever seen. I handed her to my husband for I knew he was anxious to hold her too. Although she was barely three weeks old she looked up and smiled at us, as if she sensed our uneasiness. She has maintained that ability to put people at ease. The nurse came and told me something of infant care, gave me a formula recipe, and one lone four-ounce bottle of formula. This was a bit frustrating for all the books on adoption said you were given enough formula to last for twenty-four hours. The bottle was empty before we got home. But we boiled and sterilized and after some experimentation, managed to get a batch of formula cooked up. That first week was difficult for we were afraid of this little seven pounds of femininity. But with the help of friends, the local doctor, and many phone calls to the pediatrician in Jackson, we made it. I had lost the same number of pounds that first week that our baby weighed.

I recalled that my husband's voice teacher urged him to give a recital in the late spring. He had been quite reluctant to do this and I recalled my surprise and pleasure at the way he handled the French, German, and Italian arias. I remembered the tiny red corsage he bought along with the corsages and boutonnieres he got for the usher couples, his teacher, and me. And how pretty our little three-month-old daughter looked as he showed her off to the friends who came to our house after the recital. I remembered thinking that there would doubtless be other corsages that would impress her more than the tiny red one, but none would come from a greater admirer. I remembered his dedicating one number to "A young lady who is too young to attend," and then doing Brahm's Lullaby in German.

The depressing memories had faded and happier ones were taking their place.

We spent most of Saturday outside enjoying the beautiful snow that had fallen during the night. We rode in the horse-drawn sleigh which the college owns. It was a new experience for all three of us. Later we walked to town in the snow. We had friends in for dinner. My husband made snow ice cream for dessert, for one of the guests was from the deep South and had never had snow ice cream. Life was fun again. For a while, that is.

On Saturday night I did not sleep well. Judy had developed a fever and we were worried about her. I didn't sleep much but enough to have a horrible dream. I shuddered each time I thought about it the next day. I awakened, went into another room, closed the door so the light would not disturb anyone else, and wrote it down.

The dream was about two little girls. One was around four and the other about two. The older one was playing with the younger one as if she were a doll, not realizing she was dead. It seemed that the older one was mine. I was worried about her and asked the undertaker what kind of embalming fluid he had used and whether it would hurt my little girl. I was extremely worried when my little girl picked up the dead baby. There was something about someone redressing the dead baby. I was worried about its lying so still. Sometimes it seemed as if both babies were mine. I needed some boxes for something or other. I was at my sewing machine mending a torn dress, then realized I wouldn't need it for the baby was dead. I cried in the dream and was very sad. Then there was only one child, the dead child, and it was mine.

I couldn't shake off the feeling of horror even after I had recorded the dream. I went back to bed but not to sleep. My mind was busy at work again — remembering. The feeling of depression that had left me for a few hours on Saturday had returned and brought along a companion: the feeling of horror. All day Sunday I kept recalling the dream and remembering incidents from long ago. I thought of my little sister who had died when I was about four and a half. I recalled my playmate across the road who they said was ill and I couldn't play with her anymore. I recalled not understanding this since she was not sick in bed. When I was older I learned that she had had tuberculosis and had later died. I remembered going to the spring with my older sister for a bucket of cool water and picking flowers to take to the doctor's wife who lived next door and for whom I had been named. I remembered playing with the little boy who lived down the road, and that something we did displeased my mother and that I never cared to play with him after that. That feeling had persisted: I remembered visiting my aunt who still lived in the little town, years later, and the little boy, now grown up, had wanted to take me somewhere and I wouldn't go. I remembered playing in the snow one winter's night with my older sister and two brothers, liking it and being unhappy when they took me into the house and then went out again without me. I remembered the Christmas after my little sister's death when I found so many toys under one of the beds, and being surprised that there were so many since my little sister was gone. I remembered that I hadn't told anyone about finding the toys. I remembered that my dad brought me a sack of candy every day from my grandfather's store where he worked. I remembered how I had always liked to go to Aunt Ethel's house.

All day I remembered.

I rather dreaded going to bed Sunday night. I was afraid I would have another horrible dream. I slept very little, maybe because I was worried about Judy. The doctor had come and prescribed some medication but didn't know what was causing the fever. I was up with her often but I doubt if I would have slept much anyway. I was too busy remembering. It seemed as if something was compelling me to remember everything that had ever happened to me.

When I finally got to sleep I did dream, but it did not hold the horror of the dream of the previous night. One thing seemed odd to me. I can seldom recall a dream in the morning, yet these dreams came back clearly and almost demanded to be remembered. I got up quietly, picked up my pencil and note pad, and started out of the room. My husband called to me and remarked that he didn't think I had slept long enough to dream.

But isn't it so that a dream which might cover a considerable amount of time actually takes only a few seconds to dream? I guess I had slept a few seconds, at least.

This dream had to do with needing some flowers to plant. There was something about people constructing a formal garden. But they said it was not a formal garden. It was to be a filling station. They had lots of flowers, bronze-colored mums. I wanted to get some too. They thought I might get some down the road where a playground was being torn up. Then I seemed to be on a hill that had lots of shrubbery and there were lots of people there too. I started for my car and expected Judy to follow me. When I got to my car, an old model, I realized that Judy had not followed and I was irked with her. Then I realized that she was very small and had probably gotten lost in the crowd and I was sorry that I had been irked with her. I went back to look for her.

The next morning I was tired and very depressed. Incidents kept coming back to me. Most of them I had not thought about for many years. I tried to prevent my mind's backward gazing by entertaining Judy. I wasn't able to do much about it. The need to remember seemed very strong. The day wore on and finally it was time to keep my appointment with Dr. M. and the brown leather chair.

Therapist's Summary of Session III

During the first two sessions I was, in effect, training the patient to go rapidly and deeply into hypnosis and I was also busy establishing a solid therapeutic relationship. These two factors are intimately and inseparably related. The patient reported at the third session that the intervening period had been fraught with anxiety because she had found herself preoccupied with memories from the era in question. She also believed that she had recaptured the memory for which she searched. It was the physician's remark, "The baby is dead; if we wait, she may go too" (a verbalization actually uncovered in the second session). Hypnosis was induced and the delivery scene revivified. She immediately "heard" the physician remark, "Its neck is broken." The patient identified this statement as the elusive verbalization.

She remarked upon awakening that one immediate benefit of these sessions was that for the first time she and her husband had been able to talk freely about this painful period in their lives. Even though I was yet unaware of the relationship to her primary symptom, the phobia, it became increasingly clear to me why she had brought her husband to the first session. I gathered that she felt extremely guilty about the untimely death and felt that it might have helped if the husband knew that she was not to blame in the death of their third and last child.

At the conclusion of the session, she was given the posthypnotic instruction that the meaning of her lifelong fear of dogs would begin to manifest itself between sessions. I further suggested that if these memories, thoughts, or feelings were too disturbing, they would be communicated to her in night dreams.

Session IV, Monday, February 3

It had snowed almost continuously since Sunday morning and the town looked like an old-fashioned Christmas card. But it was not the kind of weather to drive in, at least, not for me, so I called a cab to go to the state hospital. When it came, two of my students were already passengers. The driver asked where I wanted to go and I told him; one of the girls asked if I did volunteer work there. I was somewhat on the spot and finally stammered something that could be taken for an affirmative answer. I justified it to myself by thinking that what I was doing was voluntary. I couldn't tell them that their teacher was a patient at the mental hospital without some sort of explanation and I was in no mood to explain.

I went into Dr. M.'s office, sat down in the brown leather chair, and told him about the dreams. He seemed interested in them and thought it wise to investigate them more closely under hypnosis. For some reason it seemed harder for me to relax than it had been in the previous sessions. But finally I was able to let go and make my way down to the dark hallway again. Once under hypnosis it was difficult for me to relive the dreams. Something inside me seemed to rebel. Of course, Dr. M. did not force it upon me. I had to be willing. After struggling with myself for a few minutes, a little story that has helped me face many unpleasant things in my life came to keep me company and I could go on. The story was this:

Many years ago a Persian king held a birthday celebration and all the royalty from the neighboring lands came bringing gifts. There was one prince who brought a ring which he made the king promise to wear at all times before he would give it to him. The king was obviously disappointed with the gift, for it was just a simple ring which bore the words, "And even this shall pass away." As the king thought about those words he became furious with the young prince. He had everything he wanted and the inscription bothered him. Nevertheless, he wore the ring as he had promised. Then war and famine and disease came to his land. His warriors were defeated, his sons killed, and his wealth gone. All that remained was the simple ring with its inscription, "And even this shall pass away." Now for the first time the king understood the value of the gift and the wisdom of its giver.

Although I had to experience the dreams in their entirety, it was as if I were an observer rather than an actual participant, and the horror was somewhat removed. Under hypnosis the dream took on meaning, and as before, incidents that had long been sleeping took their proper places like dancers on a stage. This is what I experienced as I sat in the familiar leather chair that day.

I was a small child playing outside with my little sister and my little black dog, Rover. My two older brothers were carrying in wood from the woodpile for the stoves. My little dog and I were near the woodpile and watched as my little sister got an armful of wood just as my brothers had done and started for the house. I watched as the dog played around her and finally jumped up on her, causing her to fall. I saw my mother come and pick her up. She had fallen on the wood and scratched her face. She was crying. My mother thought I had caused her to fall and scolded me. I told her that I had not done it but she did not believe me. I told her about the dog jumping up and causing her to fall. She did not believe that either. Later that evening my mother said that we would find out who had caused my sister's fall. She had us all line up: my older sister, my two brothers, and me. Each of us was to go up to the door that opened onto the rear porch. When the guilty one got to the door there would be a rapping, she said. When I got to the door, the rapping occurred. My child's mind could not understand this, for I knew I was not guilty. Oddly enough, this door-rapping incident was something that I had consciously remembered and had asked my mother about several times. She always insisted that it had never happened. I guess she had forgotten it. But I could always remember it and remember being falsely accused of something, but I never knew what. I hadn't thought about it for many years and was surprised to find it crop up here. Looking back, I can somewhat understand why they resorted to this little game. If they were so certain that I had caused the fall, they perhaps thought the knocking would cause me to admit my guilt. But I was not guilty! As I continued to experience the dream, I was being spanked for causing my sister's fall. I was unhappy about it. I went to bed a very unhappy child. The next day, it seemed to be, my little sister was ill. In a day or two she died, apparently from the infection caused by the splinter in her cheek. There were lots of people at our house and some ladies who tried to explain death to me. All that I understood with my childish mind was that my sister was gone a long way off, to some place high up, and that if I were very good I might see her again some day. It was all confusing and the only thing I really understood was that she could not play with me anymore. While all the people were in another room I went into the room where my little sister was lying on something that resembled an ironing board. I picked her up and held her. She was very still and didn't put her arms around my neck anymore and it seemed all wrong somehow. My little dog had come into the room with me. He jumped up and accidentally tore my sister's pretty white dress. Someone, I think perhaps it was my mother, came in and was very displeased with me. She thought I had torn the dress. Someone put another dress on my sister and put her in a box — a casket, I guess — and told me not to go into the room where she was unless someone went with me. I felt very lonely after that. I did not like my dog anymore either.

My conscious mind could hardly believe what I was seeing. I had no idea that this incident had been in my life! I knew, of course, that my little sister had died. I had one or two memories connected with her death; I had heard my folks talk about it some but most of what I had been experiencing was new to me. I could recall how very much I had missed my little sister and I remembered being very disappointed a few months later when my family left the little town and moved to the city. I had expected to find my little sister there — for the ladies had told me she had gone far away and I would see her again if I were good. The city was far away (as a child reckons distance) and I had tried to be good. I can recall now that I heard my mother say in later years that the reason for moving from the little town was that the house held too many unpleasant memories for her. Was this one of them?

I was surprised to learn that I had ever been on friendly terms with a dog. I was more surprised to learn that I had, at one time, even had a dog. I can't remember what I said to the doctor or what he said to me after he awakened me. This had been a shocking experience. I was having trouble believing that it had ever really happened and wondered if my mind was playing tricks on me. I remember now that I felt confused and very lonely and that I talked to my husband about the session even before I took my coat off. I simply had trouble believing the incident could have happened and was surprised to hear him say, "Well, it makes sense to me." He went on to say that he had observed how my parents always seemed to act as if I owed them something, and that if they really thought I had caused my sister's death they perhaps felt, maybe subconsciously, that I was obligated to them. He seemed to feel that the uncovered experience could explain a lot of things. I was disappointed by his reaction, I think. I guess I had hoped he would convince me that the incident could not have happened. But by now, I was afraid it was beginning to make sense to me too. I guess I had hoped to find some unimportant little incident to account for the long-existing fear. Of course, I did not realize that an unimportant little incident probably could not have caused such a lasting fear in the first place.

I couldn't keep my mind off of the incident. Although I was beginning to accept it, it still seemed somewhat incredible. Slowly I was beginning to understand some things about my childhood, however. I was beginning to understand why I had been such a shy, withdrawn child, why I had preferred my own daydreams to the company of others, why I could never confide in my mother, yet longed to, why I had been something of a problem child, why I had often felt like an outsider and yet wanted so much to be accepted. I was also beginning to understand something else that had bothered me sometimes and made me feel a little guilty: why my husband's family had seemed closer to me than my own family had. And as I was better understanding parts of my own life, I think I was also gaining a clearer insight to some of my mother's actions. I suspect that she had been as much a victim of the incident as I had been, maybe more so. I felt sorry for her.

I was beginning to understand now why it had always been so difficult for me to discipline our little girl. I knew it was a necessary part of her training yet I was always afraid I would punish her unjustly. I told myself I felt this way because she was adopted but knew that was an excuse and not a real reason. I read the child psychology books and talked to child psychologists about this matter of discipline. I talked at great length with a pediatrician who was also a close friend. She was an ideal mother as well as a very fine doctor. She assured me that most children grow into pretty fine adults in spite of their parents, and tried to make me feel better about the discipline problem.

Also I could begin to see why I had tried so desperately to shield Judy from any associations with death. I didn't want her young mind to get any distorted ideas about death or God or any of those things. I recalled that she was four when my father had died and that I had carefully kept her away from any part of it. I couldn't understand parents who would take their young children to funeral homes and cemeteries. I knew that someday she would ask about death and I would have to try to explain it to her. I dreaded the day and thought about it a lot. I read articles about how to explain death to children and finally one day found a little story that I clipped to use when the occasion should come. Another mother had used this story to tell her children about the death of a grandmother whom they loved. This is the story:

There was a colony of bugs that lived in a murky pond on the underside of a lily pad. They noticed that every now and then one of their clan would crawl up the stem of the lily pad, disappear, and never return. This bothered them and one day they held a meeting and decided that the next one who crawled up the lily pad must promise to return and tell them what was up there. They all promised. One day one of them felt this uncontrollable urge and could not resist crawling up the stem and over the top side of the lily pad. He couldn't believe what he saw. It was such beautiful sunshine. He had never seen anything but the dark, murky water before. Then he remembered his promise. He thought and thought about it and finally convinced himself that they would not want him to leave this beautiful sunshine and go back to the murky pond, and that they would understand when their time came to crawl up the stem of the lily pad.

This was the way I had planned to present death to my child, probably because I wanted to save her from the misrepresentations I had experienced. Now I wondered if this story would be any less confusing.

I was beginning to understand why I had wanted to protect her from so many things. Of course, one cannot completely shield a child's mind, for they get ideas and impressions from so many places. I recalled one day as we were driving along the highway we were watching some interesting cloud formations. We were playing a little game — trying to make all sorts of pictures of the clouds. I recalled my surprise when Judy asked, "Mommy, if I could get on the other side of that cloud, would I see the face of God?" I never knew where she got that idea and began to realize that parents are not the only persons who plant seeds into the fertile minds of the very young.

I was beginning to understand why I stopped at nothing to insure her a happy childhood. It was almost an obsession with me. She must have happy memories of her childhood. I did not think of a happy time when I thought of my childhood but I never knew why. It was more like a big blur of unhappiness. I could not understand people who said they would like to live their childhood years again. I certainly did not want to relive mine. I was beginning to better understand why I had felt that way. I am sure there were some very happy times in my childhood but the strongest impression is one of loneliness and unhappiness.

And I was feeling lonelier now, since this last session, than I could ever remember feeling before. This feeling was much more intense than the depressing feelings which the previous sessions had caused. I kept thinking about this last visit to the state hospital and had trouble keeping my mind on my household duties and schoolwork. I got dinner over and we watched TV but I could not keep my mind on the programs. I was recalling my childhood memories instead.

Before retiring I made sure my pencil and note pad were beside my bed and wondered what horrible dream I would have to write down. But I did not dream.

I had an early class next morning, and as I walked across the campus I found myself hoping I would meet a dog. I wanted to see if my reactions would be any different, if my fear would be less intense. Although there are usually several dogs playing around the campus, I did not see one that morning. I had trouble keeping my mind on the work my class was doing and was glad when the bell rang. I felt so lonely I wanted to get away from my students as quickly as possible. I usually stop at the infirmary to say hello to the nurse but I did not want to see anyone that morning. I was in no mood to give a cheerful hello to anybody. As I neared the edge of the campus I saw a large Collie. I slowed down and he came toward me. I was surprised that I was not afraid and actually wanted him to come over to me; I patted him and was not afraid. For the first time that I could remember, I patted a dog and was not afraid! I felt that this was proof that the incident of yesterday's session was the real cause of my fear of dogs. However, as I was patting the Collie another dog, perhaps baffled at my actions, came running toward me and the old fear returned. I recoiled and found myself reacting as I had always done before, but for a few brief minutes I had been free of the fear! I could hardly wait to get home and tell my husband and daughter. But if the fear had left me for a moment, the feeling of sadness had not.

I decided to write to my mother and ask her some specific questions about the incident that seemed to account for my phobia. She was not well and had not written to me for several months, but I decided to send the questions anyway. My husband thought she would not likely reply, even if she remembered. But I sent the letter and waited. After I had written the letter I watched Judy as she sat on a window seat amused at some squirrels playing in a tree outside. I decided to sketch her. It was her birthday and she made an interesting study as she watched the squirrels. Then, too, I thought sketching her might force the lonely feeling away for a while. But I was wrong. It even splashed over onto the sketch paper — and though I could catch the feature likeness of our little girl, her happy expression eluded me and the expression of a sad child took its place. After several attempts I gave up. I could not sketch my child's happy expression. [See drawing facing p. 79.]

This had been the day for Judy's birthday party. The guests had been invited and the cake baked. There had been a party on her birthday every year before but this one had to be postponed because she was ill. I was rather glad it had been postponed for I could not have been a very cheerful hostess to her friends today. I had considered myself a rather happy individual but the events of the past two weeks made me wonder.

Tuesday night I went to bed, read a long while, and finally got to sleep. Sometime before one-thirty I awakened. I had dreamed something about several people but it was so vague that I could not recall anymore about it. Although I could not recall the dream, my mind was busy recalling events and I lay awake until around four-thirty thinking about them. I seemed compelled to write them down so I got up, took my pencil and note pad into another room, and wrote them down. I was thinking about events connected with the loss of our first baby: how it had been born just before the doctor got to our house; of the ambulance trip to the hospital; of waiting in the operating room while they worked on the baby in another room; my disappointment when the doctor said it hadn't lived and my resentment at learning that the nurse or whoever was responsible had failed to warm up the incubator as the doctor had requested on the phone. I thought about incidents surrounding my father's death: how I had left the hospital in August knowing I would not see him alive again and of my little girl's concern because I could not help crying after I got into the car. I recalled an incident just before I had lost the first baby when I couldn't get my car out of the garage, and that I was irked because my father didn't leave his grocery store and help me. I recalled that when my husband had been drafted, he had left the car with my parents and although I had driven very little I decided to use the car anyway. I recalled Dad's having an appointment with the doctor a day or two after my husband left.

I told him I would drive him to the doctor if he wasn't afraid to ride with me. He did not drive and seemed less afraid than I was. I recalled that I had to turn left into a very busy street and finally made it. I didn't know how to park a car and spent the whole time he was seeing the doctor trying to park. I made it just as he came out of the doctor's office. My recollections seemed to go back in some sort of chronological order.

I recalled the summer of 1939. I went home to help my dad in the store while Preston went on to the university to begin his graduate work, line up living quarters and, we hoped, a job for me. I vaguely recalled something about being unhappy because Dad objected to my talking to the young brother of the storekeeper across the street. There seemed to be something about golf being involved. This was such a long-forgotten memory, if there at all, and so vague that neither my husband nor I could actually recall it.

I then thought about my last year of college and events connected with it. I recalled that I was nearly expelled because of an unusual set of circumstances and was blamed for something I had not done. I was editor of the campus news sheet, the *Ghost*, partly because I enjoyed it but more because the small stipend supplemented a low family income. During a short illness someone else had edited the paper and had included an article from the question box which condemned the actions of the president's son as being very childish. All of us who knew about the incident felt that another student would have been severely punished. Had I been handling that particular issue I might have also included the contributed article from the question box. The article had been signed but the name was withheld from the paper. When the president saw the paper he was furious and stormed into our apartment without waiting to be invited and demanded to know where the article had come from. I refused to tell him, for it had come from the college nurse and I knew he would fire her on the spot. He was that angry. He knew I had not edited the sheet for I had been ill in bed with a cold. He demanded to know who had been handling it for me. He said he would expel me from school if I refused to tell him. I had to refuse to tell him. I did not have to graduate but we did have to eat and my husband, then a young teacher, had been doing the editing for me. The president was very angry and began at once to take steps to effect my dismissal. Some of the wiser administrators, and one who is still a good friend of ours, persuaded him to suspend the *Ghost* instead of its editors. To this day I do not know how the students managed to suspend such a real-looking ghost from the highest chandelier in the auditorium, but it was there the next morning for convocation. It didn't help any that the guest speaker for that morning was someone whom the president wanted to impress. I had not thought about this incident for years but it came back in clear detail. Some others did too and some returned only vaguely.

I remembered reading Lin Yutang's *The Importance of Living* three times but I couldn't remember why. I seemed to recall that I had finally graduated with honors. I wasn't sure of that. It seemed so but I could not recall it vividly. Neither could my husband when I asked him about it the next morning.

My mind then went back to a spring day during my second year at college. The student body was divided into three groups called literary societies, although the competition was in various phases of college life. The society to which I belonged had won its share of honors and I was defending our women's singles tennis title. I was doing all right and had won the first set 14-12 and was ahead on the second set when my "steady" stopped watching the match and started playing on an adjoining court with the prettiest girl in school. Of course, I was worried. I probably would have worried even if I hadn't had an inferiority complex. I like to think I was only worried but I would not like to have the feeling analyzed lest it have to be called by an uglier name. Anyhow, I lost the match — the tennis match, that is.

My mind then took a big leap back through the years to a time when I was about eight or nine. My folks had gotten me a tiny puppy, thinking, perhaps, it would help me get over my fear of dogs. There was something about washing the front porch and my younger sister being with me. The dog came onto the porch, then ran out of the yard to a neighbor's yard where it died. I had mixed emotions about its death: a feeling of relief, mostly, I think, because it was not around anymore. But I was sorry too.

I then recalled an incident that took place about the same time. My sister, about six years younger than I, had fallen down the basement stairs. My mother accused me of pushing her and I was quite unhappy about it. I hadn't thought about that incident for years but I guess it was a rather serious fall for my sister still has a concave spot high on her forehead. I had not pushed her, but if Mother still blamed me for my other sister's death maybe it was natural to think I had caused Wilma to fall too.

My memory took me still further back. I was a small child being held in some adult's arms and a dog was jumping around their feet. It was vague. Some of these memories I could not verify. But I knew there were ways to check up on some of the others and I knew I would have to do it the next day.

It was already the next day, for the last time I looked at my watch, it was 4:15 A.M. Sometime after that I dreamed a terrifying dream.

I was sitting on a low porch and a very large and ugly dog was viciously attacking me. It was biting me and knocking me over. In the dream I was surprised that I was not telling the dog to "go away" but instead was trying to quiet it. But I was so terribly afraid of it that I was trembling. I finally got the dog quieted and awakened to find myself saying, "Down, boy, down, down." After this dream the lonely feeling started gradually to disappear. It was rather like watching the morning mists or fog rise up from the valleys to a mountaintop. A happier, sunnier feeling was coming to me.

I was rather tired next morning and at breakfast asked my husband if he thought I would have to remember everything that had ever happened to me. He facetiously asked if I had yet remembered a certain light green dress that he had liked during our courting days. I hadn't, but oddly enough, immediately all the dresses that had ever held any special significance for me started parading before my mind's eye. It was almost as if someone had pulled out a drawer marked "dresses." I wondered if our minds have some sort of unique cataloging system whereby similar incidents are filed away in some sort of systematic manner.

I had to spend this day checking up on some of the half-remembered incidents that had kept me from sleeping and I had to find out what fascination Lin Yutang had held for me. I seemed compelled to do this checking even though I really could not spare the time. This was Wednesday and on Friday I was giving a bridal shower — the biggest party I had given for some time — and there was yet much to do. But I seemed unable to postpone the checking. It seemed more important than the party.

My husband is a very orderly person. He confuses me every now and then by arranging my spice shelf in such alphabetical order that I can't find a thing. He has always kept a family diary. He spent most of his spare time one winter arranging all our letters to each other in chronological order. I was fairly certain I could check the incident about the storekeeper's brother for if it were important enought to demand being remembered, it would surely appear in some of the letters. So I found the trunk that we had affectionately called "Judy's Educational Policy" (if we were not around to send her to college, she could publish our letters) and found the letters for the summer of 1939. Sure enough, there it was in a letter from me dated July 19. "I have a newly acquired friend. A young St. Louis University student came into the store and we have become good friends. He is Catholic, majoring in history, likes to read, enjoys opera and is very gentlemanly. A real find in this neighborhood. He loaned me two books last night. He would like to read our Andrew Jackson, may I loan it? He is a good conversationalist, about twenty years old. You will enjoy knowing him." Although this letter made me remember the incident quite clearly, there was nothing about golf and that had seemed rather definite in the memory. So I read some letters. In fact I spent much too much time reading even after I found what I was looking for. A letter with a later postmark contained the following: " . . . would you like to buy some golf clubs? My young friend plays golf. I mentioned that someday you and I were going to learn the game. He suggested that he teach me right now and we would make it a foursome if I wanted to take someone along — Mother or somebody. I told him that since you would also like to learn that we would wait until you returned to make it a foursome. A friend of his has a complete set of clubs that were pawned to him and since he is not a golfer he would sell the whole business for $5." We did not buy the clubs. Those were depression days and $5 was a lot of money. After finding this incident we were amused, however, at missing the bargain, for my husband gave me golf clubs for Christmas this year.

I could now clearly remember all the details of the summer. I had rather strongly resented my father's objections to my young friend. From my viewpoint it was a perfectly harmless relationship, and, of course, I was too young to see it from my father's point of view. Looking back, I can better appreciate his actions. He really had my interests at heart and was concerned lest the neighbors misunderstand.

Now that I had cleared up this recollection I had to verify the bit about graduating with honors. Actually, I doubted that I had. I found all sorts of certificates and diplomas that we had acquired but I could not find the diploma I was searching for. I called my husband's office. He had it there but said there was no indication of the honor in question. But I still felt compelled to check further. I finally found all my transcripts, and after listing all my grades pertaining to that degree, I called my husband again. Since evaluating grades is part of his routine duties, it was easy for him to check this for me. In a minute or two he said, "Yes, this appears to be an honors system." I am not sure why it was so important to find out unless it tied in with the disappointment I had felt when none of my family came to my graduation. Their failing to come was not too surprising, for they had not encouraged my going to college, or to high school either, for that matter. But they were not to be censured for that. No one in our neighborhood went to college, and very few ever started high school. Girls were expected to marry young and settle down to maintaining a home. Perhaps they had been disappointed in my delayed conformancy.

I kept thinking about Lin Yutang's book. I could not remember why it had seemed so important to me. At a faculty coffee hour on Thursday morning I talked to two of our older professors and asked if they were familiar with the book. One, whose sister had lived in China, had sent him the book but he had read only parts of it. He said I had probably been fascinated with the "chaste and beautiful" English that the writer had used. The other gentleman explained that the "mystic manner" of the book had perhaps intrigued me. I did not tell them why I had again become so interested in the book, but their answers did not satisfy and I knew I had to read it again.

I finally found a copy of the book in the college library. I was anxious to get into it, but there was a luncheon with the trustees' wives, then a class to be taught, and then it was time for my appointment with Dr. M.

Therapist's Summary of Session IV

The patient reported the following dreams (this session is transcribed, pp. 91–129, and is also on the published tape in its entirety). The first dream was about two little girls. One child was playing with the other as if she were a doll. She didn't realize the girl was actually dead. Then there was something about redressing the dead baby, and then the patient was at her sewing machine mending a badly torn dress. "Suddenly I realized my child was dead and I cried a lot in my dream. Then it seemed there was only one child, the dead one, and it was mine. It was a very sad and depressing dream. I never had a dream like that before. It was horrible even when I thought of it in the daytime."

The second dream concerned a group of people with flowers who were constructing a formal garden. There was some confusion about it being transformed into a filling station. Judy was with the patient. When she went back to her car, she suddenly found that Judy was missing. The patient was at first angry but this reaction was replaced by a feeling of being sorry that she had become irritated over the daughter's disappearance and she went to look for her. This dream was not as disturbing as the first nightmare.

In relation to the first dream, the patient volunteered, "Oddly enough when I woke from that horrible dream, I recalled my little sister's death, and I haven't thought of that for many, many years. I recall practically nothing about it. It is so long ago I just never think about that. . . . It must have been about 41 years ago, [when] I was about four." Other associations were not immediately forthcoming, so hypnosis was induced, and most of the hour was spent in allowing the full meaning of the dream to emerge.

For a 10-minute period, the patient sat in silent contemplation and then, at my prompting, she began to share a flood of memories which she apparently had repressed since childhood. She had been playing in the back yard of their home with her younger sister when the family dog, Rover, knocked the little girl down. The sister suffered a splinter wound in her cheek. Several days later the little girl died, apparently of an infection, and the mother openly blamed the patient, accusing her of knocking her sister down.

The patient next recalled the day of the funeral in some detail, particularly an incident which added to the traumatic impact of the whole situation; the same little black dog had leaped up and torn the sister's dress, and again the patient felt that she was blamed for the situation. The patient had the impression that within a short period of time, the grandfather took Rover to keep. Prior to awakening, the patient was given instructions to the effect that she was free to remember as much of this experience as she was prepared to accept. Upon awakening, she obviously recalled the entire episode.

There was not time to analyze the second dream in detail, although the patient did say under hypnosis that it dealt with the death of her older sister, and one gathers from her associations that her dying made death more palatable to the patient. I now felt that we knew the causal agent in the patient's phobia. At the conclusion of the session, a post-hypnotic suggestion was given that in the interim, the meaning of this experience and its total effect upon her life, past and present, would begin to make itself evident to her. The patient also expressed an intention to write her mother and discuss the event that therapy had uncovered.

Session V, Thursday, February 6

I made myself comfortable in the brown leather chair that had become so familiar to me and told Dr. M. what had been happening to me since I had seen him last. I remember thinking that it had become very easy to talk to him and yet if I were to meet him outside the office I wasn't sure I would recognize him. I thought about that some and decided he was easy to talk to because he was such a good listener (maybe I had learned something very important) and that I might not recognize him outside the office because I really saw him very little, since during most of our time together I was under hypnosis.

I told him about my failure to sketch my happy little girl and about my momentary freedom from the fear. I think I told him that my husband thought the incident about my little sister's death made sense to him. I told him about the book. I was a bit disappointed that he was not familiar with it. I guess I had hoped he would know what spell it had held over me. He did say, "Maybe I can help you with it." I took this to mean that he would probably read the book and help me understand why it had interested me so. That is not what he meant at all.

Dr. M. thought we should investigate the dream about the dog with the ugly face. I was not too anxious to re-experience it but we finally made our way down the dark hallway, past the door on the left until we came to a place that seemed new to me. From where we were there appeared to be the end of the hallway and daylight, or some kind of light, at the far end. It was like approaching the end of a mountain tunnel. The dream seemed not to come from any actual experience in my life and I hoped it might be symbolic of my struggle with the fear, and that I was finally going to defeat it.

Then Dr. M. said we would look at the book. He asked me to picture it and said the leaves would turn as if being blown by a breeze and would stop at a significant page. This actually seemed to happen. When the breeze stopped the page did contain a phrase that seemed to be significant, yet it puzzled me. I seemed to see clearly Shakespeare's words, "To thine own self be true." I wondered if some mysterious trickster had slipped the wrong book into my hand. I knew I had to read the book again to learn whether it actually contained these words.

I believe I also re-experienced a previous dream and some previous thoughts that had seemed important, but generally memory of the session was vague. Before Dr. M. awakened me he asked if there was anything else I wanted to talk about. I told him I had a dental appointment for the following Monday morning, and since I had always more or less dreaded a trip to the dentist I thought it would be an interesting experience to see whether hypnosis might also work here. I asked if he thought he could make me less sensitive to the vibrations caused by the drill. I did not ask him to take the pain away for I always had novocaine anyhow and would surely use it for this cavity since an X-ray had revealed it to be a rather bad one. Dr. M. asked if this was something I wanted very much to do. I assured him that it was. And he proceeded to give me the necessary suggestion. He must have told me not to remember the suggestion when I awakened for I can't seem to recall what he really said.

I left the office feeling better than I had for quite a while. My mind was not free from its remembering but I was beginning to feel more like a happy person again. There were times during the past two weeks when I wasn't sure whether I was a very normal personality after all. I knew that for the time, at least, I was not a happy one.

I was anxious to get to the book. I intended to read it again, for now I had two reasons for doing so: I had to find out what my original interest had been and I had to learn whether that Shakespearean quotation was really there.

I was busy that evening for my co-hostess and I were making final preparations for the bridal shower which was to be the next evening. We prepared the large filled angel cakes and other foods, which she generously sampled and wondered why I did not. Although I had lost much of the depression and was happier, my appetite had not yet returned. We worked until quite late and sometime after midnight I got into bed, adjusted my reading lamp and began, for the fourth time, to read Lin Yutang's *The Importance of Living.*

First, I checked the index for all the Shakespearean quotations. The one I sought was not there. I was disappointed but thought it might have accidentally been omitted from the cross reference. I then decided to start searching for it page by page. The book was interesting. I could see what my professor-friend had meant about the "chaste" English. I could also understand what the other professor meant too. There was something of the Confucian philosophy, and something rather mysterious that he called the Laotsean outlook. There was the philosophy of the Christian and the pagan. It was all very interesting. I had read about an hour when I found something in the chapter entitled "Find Thyself" that interested me particularly. It dealt with a philosophy which the author called the "half-and-half" or the average Chinaman's religion. The conflict between action and inaction, ending in compromise or contentment with a very imperfect heaven or earth, gave rise, he said, to a wise and merry philosophy of living. He went on to say, "The only problem unconsciously assumed by the Chinese philosophers to be of any importance is: How shall we enjoy life, and who can best enjoy life? No perfectionism, no straining after the unattainable, no postulating of the unknowable, but taking poor, mortal human nature as it is, how shall we organize our life that we can work peacefully, endure nobly and live happily?"

I was so interested that I continued to read for several hours. I was interested in his views about religion and remembered that the college I had attended had been definitely denominational, and had, quite naturally, stressed its own particular viewpoint which I had resisted their efforts to indoctrinate. While there I had learned to appreciate the lines from Tennyson's "In Memoriam" which said, "There lives more faith in honest doubt, believe me, than in half the creeds."

I read on and on without finding the quotation that I was looking for. However, as I neared the end of the book I found something that seemed to sum up my interest in the book. It also contained the very essence of the Shakespearean quotation. It said, "Religion, or peace of mind, or happiness or whatever you want to call it, is but being sincere with oneself and with the universe. . . . No one can be natural and happy unless he is intellectually sincere with himself." Hadn't the Shakespearean quotation meant exactly the same thing in *Hamlet* where Polonius says "This above all — to thine own self be true; and it must follow, as the night the day, thou canst not then be false to any man"? To me, an interesting sidelight to this is that on February 16, about two weeks later, Dr. Carl R. Rogers, a psychologist appearing on the "Wide, Wide World," TV program said, "Most of man's troubles come when he fails to do as Shakespeare has suggested, 'To thine own self be true.' "

Sometime later I turned off the light and fell asleep immediately.

My husband and daughter awakened before I did and were surprised to find me still asleep. During the past few weeks I was always awake quite early. When I did awaken they urged me to stay in bed and rest, and I was tempted to, but remembered that this was the day for the shower and reluctantly declined their offer.

It seemed as if I had been given a reprieve from remembering. My mind was free to attend to the party plans. I really hadn't been able to give much thought to them before, but now I was even able to come up with some unusual decorating ideas. I managed, with the help of my cleaning lady, to get everything done and have enought time for a luxurious bath before dressing. I had bought a new dress for the occasion three or four weeks ago. It had been slightly tighter than I like when I bought it and I was surprised at the way it fit now. There seemed to be inches to spare. I knew I had been losing some weight but a check on the bathroom scales revealed a loss of about thirteen pounds.

The party seemed to be a success. The main topic of conversation, however, was not about the beautiful gifts that the bride-to-be received, but rather about my weight. Comments ranged from envy to concern. Most of the guests saw me only at school where I wore my work smock which concealed my lost weight. The new dress did not, and to a group of such diet- and figure-conscious females the smaller waistline was bound to cause comment. And just last week someone said they were glad to see me looking better, that a couple of weeks ago they thought I had looked ill. I did not tell them that reliving the past can make one feel ill sometimes.

Some of the women urged me to tell them what reducing method I had used. I could only tell them it was not a method I would recommend to my friends. A day or two earlier some of my students wanted the same information.

After the guests had all gone and the necessary straightening up had been done, I was very tired and dreamless sleep was very welcome that night. I was still tired when I awakened the next morning. I rested most of the day and then the remembering started all over again. At one meal that day I was talking to my husband about all the remembering I had been doing. He asked if I really thought my memory was better, then with a mischievous twinkle in his eye reminded me that he had actually asked for milk to drink but I had given him iced tea. But if I were more absent-minded than usual, I certainly was better on the remembering business.

The things I kept remembering now I didn't want to discuss with Dr. M. In the first place it seemed rather silly to have to remember these incidents for they seemed to have no apparent connection with the main purpose of my visits to the state hospital. In the second place, even though it had become easy to talk to Dr. M., I did not want to discuss this side of my life. I talked to my husband about these recollections and he teasingly said, "Well, you can't keep Dr. Freud out of all this, you know." The remembering now seemed to deal with the male interest, or rather lack of male interest, in my life. In the first place, there had not been a serious interest until I met my husband and in the second place, much of the remembering had to do with male friends and acquaintances with whom, or about whom, there had not been even the slightest suggestion of a romantic interest. So I didn't see that "Dr. Freud" had any real interest in the matter.

The remembering seemed to follow the usual pattern of chronology. The first memory concerned the night of May 12, about six years ago. I was to undergo major surgery the next morning and was apprehensive about it. It was about midnight and I was still reading when one of our doctor-friends stuck his head into my room to learn why my light was still on. He had been called for an emergency and just happened to pass my room. His manner was kind, but it was also firm when he told me he wouldn't operate on me the next morning if I didn't go to sleep. I told him I didn't want him to operate on me if he didn't go home and get some sleep, that he had to be wide awake tomorrow and I didn't. He said he would order me a stronger sedative and that I could do lots of reading in a few days. I told him I was nearly finished and wanted to find out how the book ended just in case he was not as good a doctor as I thought. We kidded about it. Perhaps he knew I was trying to hide my fear. He said I might finish the book if I would promise to call the nurse as soon as I got to the last page. I did. She brought me the sleep that he had ordered. It was welcome. I could not have gone to sleep without it. I was very much afraid. My sister had not survived surgery a few years ago and I was now the same age she had been then. Perhaps I felt a bit superstitious. Next morning as I was going into surgery I told my husband I hoped he'd enjoy the floor show, for I knew he planned to watch the operation. I tried to be casual, but I was actually afraid.

I recalled several other incidents. Then I think I remembered every date that I had ever had. I had completely forgotten about some of them. I was surprised that there were as many as there were. I recalled that someone in my family would invariably tease me and I would no longer be interested. It was quite a while before I could enjoy the give and take of teasing. I remembered a proposal that I had not been happy about at the time. Looking back, I think I should have been grateful, for every woman likes to remember that there was at least one other chance.

I recalled the first night my husband walked home from church with me. He was our choir director as well as youth director. I sang in the choir. During the prayer he handed me a note. After reading it I was a bit puzzled. He had also handed a note to the girl sitting beside me. My note had asked if he might walk home with me. After a while the girl next to me whispered, "Which night does he want you to direct the youth service? " I rather liked this clever young man and even my family's teasings did not dull my interest.

I even recalled the boys I had known in high school and grade school. I remembered the Christmas when I was thirteen. A boy gave me a box of candy and some pearls. I did not want to show these to my parents lest they disapprove. This was the same boy who had written me a note some weeks earlier that my mother had scolded me and my brothers teased me about. So naturally I did not want them to know about the gifts. Looking back, however, I rather wonder where he got the pearls. I still have them.

I recalled other boys in grade school and how my brothers, and the rest of the family for that matter, teased me and I did not like it. I am sure I was an oversensitive child. Maybe these experiences have made it possible for me to better understand my little daughter, though. She talks very freely to me about her many boyfriends at school and has a free and easy relationship with them. A day or two ago she told me she was trying to persuade one of them to be her cousin and then proceeded to ask me what cousin meant. I think she is fickle, however, for she changes boyfriends quite often and has many at the same time. But at nine, that is probably permissible.

I then recalled a couple of incidents that had been long forgotten. I remembered that I had wanted to talk to my mother about them and had not been able to. Now, I think I know why I could not. One had to do with the young boarder who shared my brother's room and the other with a dentist in the neighborhood. I did not like their attentions, which I was too young to fully understand, and I wanted to talk to my mother about it. I recall that I was worried but fortunately handled the situations by myself. I recalled, however, that I caused a mild family scene when I refused to visit the dentist's office alone again. Had I been able to explain, my mother would certainly have understood.

My mind then went back to a time when I was about seven. We lived upstairs in a two-family flat. The downstairs was temporarily empty and I was playing down there with my two brothers and a friend of theirs. I was very frightened when the friend pulled me into a dark closet. I do not recall that I was harmed in any way but I was frightened and wanted to tell my mother about the incident, but could not. Because of these things, I have tried very hard to keep the relationship between my little daughter and me such that she can tell me anything. Thus far, I think I have succeeded.

All day Sunday I kept recalling these things that I did not want to discuss with my doctor. I did not sleep well Sunday night, partly because I was afraid I would have another horrible dream, but mostly, I think, I was devising ways to hide these recollections from Dr. M.

Monday brought two appointments: one with the dentist in the morning and one with the brown leather chair in the afternoon.

During the weekend I had found myself being rather anxious for Monday morning to arrive. That seemed odd. I had never looked forward with any enthusiasm to a previous dental appointment. My appointment was for nine. I was surprised to find myself wondering if I might like to try it without novocaine. Then I recalled the previous cavity just two weeks before, which had not only caused discomfort at the time of filling but had hurt for several days afterward. And I had had novocaine with that one.

When I got into the dentist's office and sat down in the chair I saw that the syringe was already filled and lay on the white towel just waiting for me. When the dentist came in he said, "I guess we had better deaden it." To which I replied, "Well, I don't know." He looked at me a bit puzzled and said, "You wouldn't want to try it without deadening it, would you? " He really looked puzzled when I said after a minute's hesitation, "Yes, let's do try it that way." Frankly, I was surprised at myself too.

He kept grinding and grinding with his new diamond drill, the same one that he had previously used, while the nurse kept water flowing into the tooth. And I felt no pain. Nor was I aware of the vibrations that had bothered me so much before that the dentist said he would not like to have to do much drilling on my teeth. When the grinding was finally finished, the dentist looked at me carefully and asked if I really felt all right. I assured him that I felt fine and asked if the cavity had been very bad. He replied that it really had been a bad one and suggested that I touch it with my tongue and see for myself. Only the tooth's shell remained. Obviously it had been a bad cavity. But I had felt no pain.

The dentist seemed quite surprised. I was one of his patients who had deserved no medals for bravery in his chair. He asked what I had been doing, if I had been using Yoga on myself. I did not tell him of the hypnotic suggestion of the previous Thursday. I did tell him to remind me to tell him all about it someday — that I thought he would be interested. He may have to read this to learn my little secret of that day.

I sat in the dentist's chair, unable to concentrate on what he was doing. Rather I was enjoying some very pleasant memories. Later, I couldn't help but think what a boon to the medical profession hypnosis could be and to wonder if, in the not-too-distant future, it might not be able to replace a lot of the anesthetics that are so necessary today. I wondered if, in another generation or two, when it was fully understood and accepted, it would not go a long way toward solving most of man's problems, mental and physical as well, and take its place along with the other great discoveries of the century.

After the dental appointment I went directly to my husband's office for I was anxious to tell him about it. I think it was difficult for him to believe that I had actually felt no pain, but he seemed obviously pleased. We had lunch together. He was surprised at that. I had not been able to eat either lunch or dinner after my previous trip to the dentist.

Therapist's Summary of Session V

At the beginning of the fifth session, the patient volunteered, "If there is any question about our making progress, we are." She stated that for the first time in her (adult) life, she had petted a dog (refer to pp. 129–130). She also reported a reassuring dream in which she was attacked by a large, vicious dog but managed to calm him.

In the three days between sessions, the patient had experienced the compulsive recall of a series of memories beginning in the recent past and extending back to early childhood. In the waking state and under hypnosis, these experiences were explored in detail. Through them ran a theme of feeling misunderstood and mistreated by her family, strong resentment and associated guilt, and a continuous struggle for independence and self-realization.

One memory concerned an event at age eight involving a puppy her parents gave her in hopes she would overcome her fear. She reported in detail an episode in which she feared the dog might attack another younger sister, and how immediately afterward, it had a fit and died. This experience apparently reinforced the potency of the original trauma.

Careful exploration revealed that the patient seemed to have no conscious knowledge of the reason underlying her intense fear of dogs, even at this age. The patient subsequently was regressed to successive age levels, but no evidence whatsoever could be found to indicate that she had ever experienced a physical attack by a dog which would account for her fear. This indirectly testified to the validity of the early experience recalled in the previous session in establishing her phobia.

The patient, incidentally, had been able to verify many of her recently recovered memories pertaining to the past 20 years by reference to a meticulous, daily family diary and file of all letters they had ever exchanged, kept by her husband. A posthypnotic suggestion again was given that the full meaning and effect of this early experience would continue to manifest itself. In addition, she asked that I give her a posthypnotic suggestion that would rid her of all pain at a forthcoming appointment with the dentist.

Session VI, Monday, February 10

I kept my appointment with Dr. M. I had no dreams to report, but I told him about my dental experience. I gave him the sketch of Judy that he had asked to see and we talked for a while. He asked whether I had told anyone about my trips to the state hospital. I told him that my husband had talked some to our president and business manager about it. They are good friends as well as associates. I told him I had talked to the college nurse about it, but he already knew that. He said that people would naturally wonder why they saw me coming there regularly. I assured him that I had no objections to anyone knowing why I went there. Later, it dawned upon me that I would prefer that they know *exactly* why I went there rather than to wonder.

This session was spent in an effort to find out whether there were any other incidents in my life concerned with dogs that might have a bearing on the fear. There seemed to be none. Apparently the doctor had found the cause of the disease. Finally he awakened me on the familiar letter. We talked about something or other, maybe about my disappointment at not losing the entire fear all at once. Then something happened that upset me and I wondered if I really were a normal individual after all.

I glanced over to the corner where the wash basin stood and thought I saw a small black dog sitting there. My conscious mind told me it could not be and yet it was there: the same little black dog that I had seen in the incident concerning my sister's death. The little dog named Rover. He seemed to be looking at me with a sort of hurt expression and I felt sorry for him. I felt confused and wondered if this phobia wasn't worse than I had thought. I reluctantly told Dr. M. about it. He didn't help much. He acted as if it were a natural thing to expect. He did not assure me that I had not seen it. Now I was confused. I recalled that one is supposed to humor the mentally ill who think they see things that aren't there and that is exactly what Dr. M. was doing with me. So we talked about Rover. He asked if I wouldn't like to take the dog home with me. It all seemed sort of foolish, but oddly enough I felt as if I really would like to take him home with me. So Rover and a very confused patient left the Clinic Building that day.

Rover seemed really to be with me and I found myself glad for his company. I found that I thought about him a lot in my spare time when I was alone and even imagined that I held him on my lap and patted him. My whole mental attitude toward dogs seemed to be undergoing a change. Maybe Rover had to be with me in order to help me accomplish this. After all, he had apparently caused the trouble in the first place, so it was only fair that he help me get out of it.

One incident occurred the next day which indicated a new pattern of thinking: I had carved most all the meat from a ham bone and my husband said he would take it out to the incinerator if I would wrap it. He laughed when I objected and said I would give it to one of the neighborhood dogs instead. I kept thinking about dogs more and more, and with a new feeling toward them, and finally it was the day for Rover and me to keep our appointment with Dr. M.

I had about given up hope of hearing from my mother. I knew she did not feel well, and though I have always written to her once every week, she had not written to me for months. But today a letter from my sister came. It contained the answers to the questions I had sent Mother. Nothing was confirmed except the fact that there had actually been, at the time of my little sister's death, a little black dog. My conscious memory had had no recollection of it. Mother said the dog did not belong to me but to my brother. That did not bother me, for possession to a four-year-old is a very vague thing. She said the dog was named Twister and not Rover. That bothered me a little. But the fact that there had actually been a little black dog was confirmation that my mind was not just creating a story. Then, too, she might have forgotten the other things, or maybe they had been erased from her mind as they had been from mine. But she did verify the existence of a little black dog!

I was pleased that I seemed to be returning to a happier state of mind. The depression was about all gone and I was beginning to feel like myself again. It was sort of like awakening from a long and restless sleep to find a beautiful new sunshiny day waiting to be enjoyed.

Therapist's Summary of Session VI

The patient appeared more relaxed than at any time since the first session. First of all she reported that the suggestion that I had given her about her dental appointment was completely effective, somewhat to her happy surprise and much to her dentist's amazement. She verbalized a number of new-found insights; for example, she now understood why she had always had the need to be liked and the fear of offending others, the basis for her deep-seated ambivalence toward her mother, and the reason underlying her discomfort in disciplining her daughter. Another insight pertained to her revulsion at touching dogs; the lively or frisky feeling of the dog brought back, through contrast, the limp feeling of her little sister experienced at the time of her funeral.

During the session the technique of age regression was again employed, and the period between her early traumatic experience and the one at age eight, uncovered in the previous session, was explored. So far as could be determined, conscious memory of the earlier event ceased to exist even prior to age five. To the end of determining what there had been in the movie *Three Faces of Eve* that finally had prompted her to seek professional help, the patient was instructed to project on an imagined movie screen the scenes from the movie which had, consciously and unconsciously, the greatest personal meaning for her. A fairly strong identification with the movie patient was revealed, based on the similarity of childhood experiences relative to death and the resulting feeling that no one, parents or spouse, seemed to understand the consequent emotional disturbance. The movie also increased her optimism that she might be helped, especially through hypnosis.

A major therapeutic tactic designed to facilitate the relearning process was introduced near the conclusion of the session. The patient was given the posthypnotic suggestion that between sessions, whenever she was alone and desired to re-establish her acquaintance with Rover, the dog of her early childhood, she could experience a positive visual hallucination of him. It was emphasized that the dog *symbolized* her disturbing history, and his fantasy relationship provided her with the opportunity to make peace with her past. It was further emphasized that she had complete control of the relationship and could "allow the dog as close as [she] desired or keep him as distant as [her] fear dictated" (refer to pp. 130–140).

Session VII, Thursday, February 18

I settled down in the brown leather chair, showed Dr. M. the letter from my mother, and we talked about Rover. I think I rather rapidly slid into hypnosis. I am not really sure what we talked about under hypnosis that day. I recall that after I awakened I felt as if I had been very deeply asleep. Maybe we talked some more about Rover, but I am not sure. He showed me a sheaf of papers which he said contained the content from these sessions; his secretary had taken it off the tapes. I expressed an interest in writing up my experience with hypnosis, for to me it had been one of the most interesting experiences of my entire life. I told him that my husband and I wanted to hear the tapes together. He suggested that I wait until I had completed my writeup. I was surprised when he said he had about nine hours of tape. I realized that I had taken a lot of a busy man's time. Rover and I left to return in about a month.

My remembering did not stop altogether. My time seemed to be divided between remembering and thinking about dogs. I found myself sort of wishing I had a little puppy. My family seemed pleased and surprised when I told them that. On Saturday I rode to a neighboring town with two friends. I was surprised when I felt as if I wanted to pet the dogs I saw in the farmhouse yards.

On Sunday night (February 16) I dreamed that a big dog jumped up on me and I was not afraid. It was more as if a child were leaning against me. Formerly I had always recoiled at the way a dog felt.

On Tuesday Judy wanted me to go to the lake with her for I had not seen her skate for quite a while and she had learned some new tricks, she said. There were three dogs playing around. A few weeks earlier this would have made me so uncomfortable that I would have fled. Instead it seemed easy and natural for me to pet the friskiest one. I was surprised that it quieted down and seemed to like the attention. I was also surprised that I did not cringe anymore at touching it. It did not feel any different from any other live object. I guess all this surprised Judy too, for I heard her yell, "Look, kids, my mother used to be afraid of dogs and she's not anymore."

After this incident Rover disappeared. I don't know whether he was jealous of the attention I had given the other dog or not. I don't know what has happened to him. But he didn't seem to be around anymore. I had trouble even thinking about him. I wondered if he will be under the wash basin waiting for me when I returned to Dr. M.'s office and I felt a little sorry that he was gone.

On the following Saturday Judy had the neighbor's puppy on the porch. This dog is so active that it must be kept on a leash, but I was not afraid to hold it while Judy put on her roller skates. I was surprised that it, too, seemed to get quiet and lie very still when I petted it.

On Sunday we went to an open house at Seminole Hall. Outside was the most interesting little black Cocker Spaniel and I felt that I would like to have one like it. As we left the hall a huge Newfoundland, a mascot of one of the fraternities, was waiting for its masters. My family asked if I didn't want to pet it. I had no objections, but I seemed to be more interested in the smaller puppies. That puzzled me some, for it had been the smaller, more active puppy that I had been most afraid of.

Tuesday, February 25, was my husband's birthday and I found myself selecting greeting cards with dog pictures on them. I got one for Judy that had five or six little puppies on it and purposely put the one back that I had first selected — it had a French poodle on it. I knew my husband would tease me about this for he had kidded me a lot about my metamorphosis.

The mail that day brought the usual things plus some birthday cards and something of great interest to me. I had asked my sister to check through the family photos and find one that had been taken a few months after my little sister's death. I could recall having the picture made and being unhappy about it. There was a dog on either side of me, and I was uneasy even though some one was holding the dogs. I could not recall what kind of dogs they were. Mostly I could remember being unhappy and afraid of having the picture made. Here was the picture. It contained two little black puppies. They looked alike and very like the little black dog in the incident that we had found under hypnosis.

My husband suggested that since there were two dogs in the picture, perhaps one had been mine and the other my brother's as Mother had remembered, that perhaps one had been called Twister and the other Rover. [Refer to photograph opposite.]

Yesterday (March 5) a phone call came for my husband. I explained that he would be out of town for the rest of the week but I would gladly take a message. The man who was calling said, "Tell your husband that I have contacted the people about the dog and it will not be available until around the first of May." As I put down the phone I had a feeling that I should not have taken that message. I did not know he was trying to locate a dog for us, but I was pleased that he apparently has confidence that I am about to lick my problem. I hope the puppy will be a little black one.

As I think back over the events of the past several weeks I feel almost as if I have been away from my usual surroundings, living another life.

Or maybe I feel like one who has completed a difficult course and has successfully studied for the examination: the loose ends are sort of tied up and satisfactory answers can be found for any question.

I have spent considerable time reflecting upon the events connected

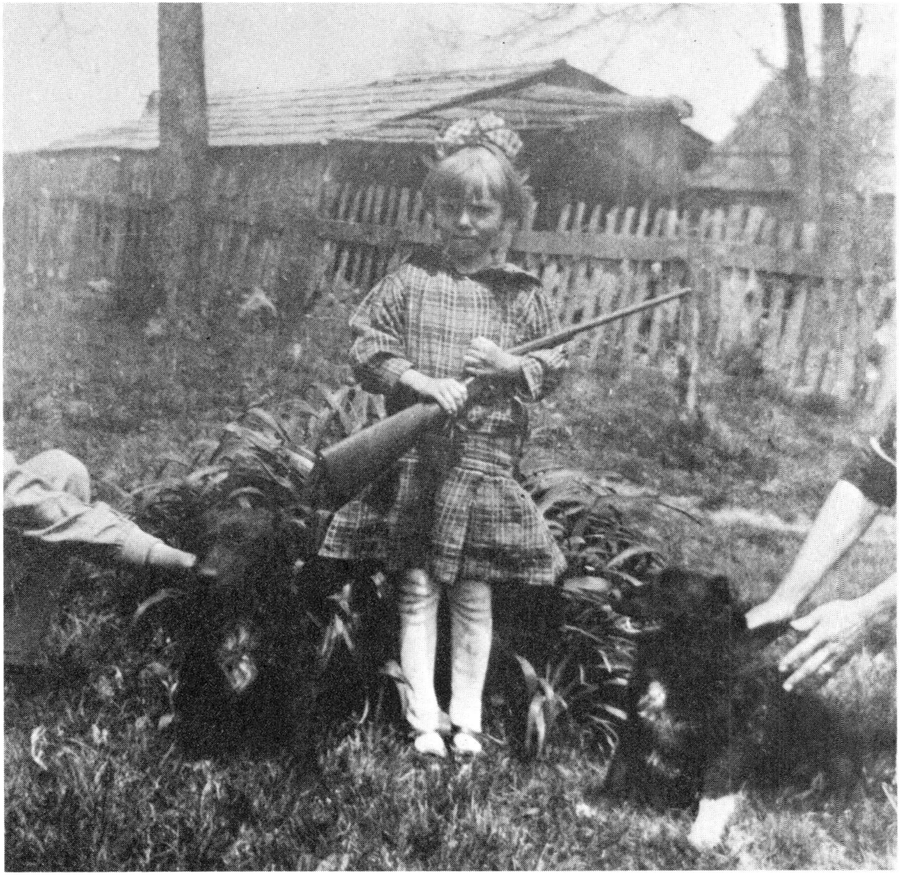

The patient at age five and a half at her grandfather's farm. The two dogs (Rover and Twister?) had to be restrained, and she felt that the gun gave her added protection.

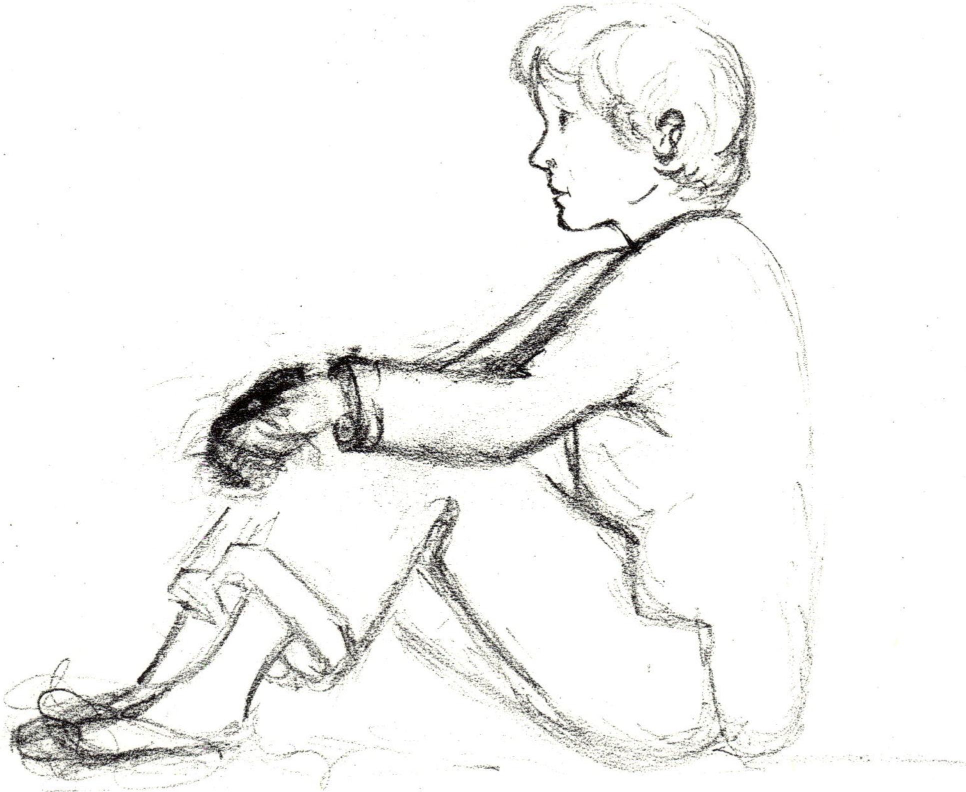

The patient's drawing of her daughter.

with the sessions in the brown leather chair. I have thought a great deal about my husband's saying he had observed my folks acting as if I owed them something. Really I think I grew up feeling obligated to them, but for a different reason. I felt that I had disrupted their lives even before I was born and had felt responsible for Mother's nearly dying when I was born. I heard them talk about Mother's ill health before my birth, of the doctor's advising them to leave their little farm and move to town where he could look after Mother constantly. I had heard them tell of leaving their little farm and buying the house next door to the doctor. I had heard them tell how I had not responded to a normal diet and of the expense involved in ordering cases of a special milk powder. I had heard them talk of how Mother nearly died and of her giving me to my Aunt Ethel because the doctor told her to decide who should raise me. I had heard them talk of my being a frail child and of the medical expense involved. And I could remember all the medicine I threw away when they were not looking. All this had probably made me feel some sort of obligation. I was freed from part of this, however, the last time I talked to Aunt Ethel. She said I had not been the cause of my mother nearly dying. There had been prenatal complications but the delivery had been normal, she said. The thing that nearly caused my mother's death took place a week later. My two older brothers had broken some windows out of a neighbor's house and since my father was not there to punish them, Mother did so from her bed. She had my older sister get a tree switch and bring the boys in and she handled the situation from there. She nearly died from the exertion for she had been suffering from a temporary heart involvement.

As I thought about my life I better understood a lot of things. Maybe I had not been a very healthy child because I was not a very happy child. They go somewhat hand in hand. I recalled having the impression that my grandfather did not like me. I was not actually aware of this myself, but rather I had gathered the impression from things I had heard. I really don't remember my grandfather too well for he died when I was quite young. If he really did dislike me, perhaps it stemmed from the incident concerning my little sister's death. I do recall hearing the folks say she had been a favorite of his. Perhaps he, too, thought I had been responsible for her death.

I thought about the lack of affection I had felt as a child. On the other hand, I doubt that I was actually aware of this as a child. It was not that my parents withheld affection from me and lavished it on the other children. It was rather that we were not an affectionate family. As I became an adult I had a very logical explanation for the fact that my parents showed a preference for my younger sister and the brother just older. After all, my sister was their baby, and my brother had the same birthday as my mother. I suspect that my parents loved their chidren just as much as other parents do; they just didn't show their affection. I think that could be explained somewhat by my mother's own childhood. Her mother died when she was very young, perhaps about a year old. She, her brother, and sisters were each taken by a different relative until Grandfather remarried sometime later. Apparently the stepmother was not happy with the responsiblity of all the children and actually had no affection for them. If my childhood was not a happy one, perhaps my mother's was even less happy.

Although I do not recall my childhood as happy, there were undoubtedly some happy times. When I try very hard I can recall family picnics in the park, vacation trips to visit Aunt Ethel, and there were the semi-annual street car trips downtown where all of us got new outfits and all sorts of unusual candies and things. It is unfortunate that the incident concerning my sister's death occurred. Perhaps my parents were hurt more than I was. Of course, they loved me. I can recall their extreme concern when I was very ill with diphtheria and when I was missing after the tornado destroyed our school building. They hadn't been able to find me because I had had to walk a long way on unfamiliar streets because of the destruction. I can recall being very happy when they gave me a complete set of oil paints when I was eleven years old.

If I do think of my childhood as an unhappy time, I feel that I have become a happier person as the years have gone by. I can think of many incidents and people who contributed to my becoming a happy individual.

I recall the two grade school teachers who spent much time with me. I wondered then why they did it. Looking back, I know. They recognized a maladjusted child in their classroom. I can recall the eighth grade teacher who took me across town and paid for lessons from an expression teacher who helped me prepare the speaking part I had in the graduation program. I recall that I wondered why I had been chosen for the part.

I recall the old gentleman who lived next door to us from the time I was about eight years old until his death some years after I was married. He was always a friend to me. He was as Catholic as my family was

Protestant and as I got older I learned to respect his religion because of him.

I recall my best friend in the neighborhood. Her mother became a very close friend too. Her mother and I would walk to the municipal opera each week during the summer while my friend was taking a special course in surgical nursing at Johns Hopkins in Baltimore. They were devout Lutherans and I learned to appreciate their faith.

I recall the Jewish family who treated me like a daughter. I had gone into their shop with a friend who wanted to buy a coat. I did not realize that I was helping to sell it to her but after the purchase, the lady asked me if I would like to work in their shop. I could not understand why she wanted me to. I was just a freshman in high school but her offer made it possible for me to complete the four years. I worked one or two evenings a week and every Saturday. Their two daughters were blonde and so was I and many salesmen thought I was the third daughter.

While in high school a whole new world opened up to me. They had an excellent art department and I took every course. I joined some clubs and held officer posts in some. I made the honor society and the glee clubs. I worked on the yearbook and the newspaper. I had parts in plays. I had lots of friends. There were three or four teachers who encouraged me to go to college. It seemed an impossible dream then, but their thinking I could gave me more confidence in myself.

I remembered the man who made and gave me my first easel. I was pleased that he thought I had some art ability. I remembered my first course in graduate school. I had been out of school for several years and was not at all sure that I could do the work that these younger students were doing. And I had a notion that graduate school was very difficult anyway. Also, I already had my hands full with household duties, a little four-year-old who needed some of my time, and my invalid mother who was living with us. I had my regular teaching duties and I had to commute forty miles to get to my graduate class. I felt as if I were undertaking the impossible but I wanted to try it. I spent every spare minute working on the course. I slept little, ate little, and lost weight. I recalled that I was mystified when I learned I had been given an A-plus for the course. But the grade was not the important thing. I knew then that I could handle the graduate work. I learned that I could work half as hard and still make acceptable grades. I thoroughly enjoyed the rest of the courses.

I recalled what it meant to both of us when my pediatrician-friend and her surgeon-husband asked if we would accept the guardianship of their four children if the need should arise. It was especially meaningful to me for it evidenced her confidence in my ability to deal with my child in spite of the worrying I had done about the matter of discipline.

I remembered the Japanese Hawaiian students who named their first child for my husband and two years later named their daughter for me. I remembered with pride the confidence they had seemed to have in us when they were in our classes.

There were many people who had helped me outgrow the frustrations of childhood and lose much of the insecurity and inferiority I had felt as an adolescent and young adult.

I know that my husband's family's complete acceptance of me has contributed greatly to my happiness. It meant a great deal to me that on one or two occasions his mother confided in me rather than her own children. His family is very close to me, and the big old home where his mother still lives, and where he was born, seems just as much my home as it does his, I am sure.

And the confidence of my child is not a small thing. I recall the night she brought her goldfish bowl with her two dead goldfish to me and wanted me to fix them. She didn't know they could not survive a bubble bath with her. Fortunately I had read that table salt will revive fish that are not too long dead and went to work on her pets. After ten or fifteen minutes of changing water and adding salt one of the fish revived. I think she thought it was a small miracle and I know I did. A child's confidence is an inspiring thing.

Of course, the one most responsible for straightening out a lot of my personality kinks is my husband. He had confidence in any abilities I had and laughed at my shyness and teased me about it until most of it has disappeared. He was patient with my fear when it must have seemed groundless and foolish to him.

And of course it was Dr. M. who so patiently helped me untangle the twisted threads, find the dropped stitches, and reweave the fabric of my life.

As I review all these things that have happened to me since my little sister's death when I was four, the thing I regret most is not the worrisome fear of dogs that seemed to stem from it, but rather my strained feelings toward my parents. I feel that both of us were cheated because of this and probably neither was fully responsible for the estrangement. I can better understand now why I was reluctant to have my mother live with us after my father's death. I remember I was proud of my husband for suggesting that she come and ashamed of myself for my lack of enthusiasm about her coming. I think I understand now.

I suspect that this early incident affected my feelings toward my younger sister and my older brothers. I always felt closer to my older sister but did not know why until these past few weeks. Apparently she had at least doubted that I had caused my little sister's fall. Although I seldom see my brothers, my younger sister and I have grown much closer during the past two or three years, in spite of the fact that our interests are widely different.

I do not know whether I have all the problems of my life solved or thought through. I do not know whether I am completely free of my fear of dogs. I seem to recall that the doctor said it might take time. I do know that I think, feel, and react differently to them.

I do not know what complexes or tendencies these sessions might have uncovered. I do not know into what category, psychologically speaking, my personality would fall. I do not know what a clinical diagnosis of this experience with hypnosis would be.

I do know that I feel that it was a very satisfying adventure. It is good to feel that my past has no secrets from me. It is also good to feel, that though the future has, they will not be revealed until the proper time.

I know that I have a sense of well being, a peace of mind, and that I am happy, maybe even happier than I have been before. I am sure that the happiness which I now have is a temporary thing, that new clouds will form on the horizon, if not now, then later. I suspect that the peace of mind is more permanent, and maybe I feel somewhat like the

Kansas statesman, William Allen White, who said: "I'm not afraid of tomorrow, for I have seen yesterday and oh, how I love today."

Therapist's Summary of Sessions VII and VIII

The patient reported that she had written to her mother concerning the recovered disturbing memories and that although the mother had confirmed the existence of a small, black dog, she insisted that the patient's fear was the result of prenatal conditioning. This seemed quite inconsistent to the patient since, from other sources, she knew that they had had several family dogs prior to the time when she was four and had never had another except for the puppy when she was eight.

The patient reported increased feelings of comfort in her general relationships with dogs. She had been able to experience Rover's hallucinated presence quite vividly and also had succeeded to some extent in making friends with him. She laughingly referred to him as "my little black Harvey." At this juncture, the patient agreed that sufficient progress had occurred to warrant a month's vacation from therapy; however, she requested that she be allowed to keep Rover in order to further renew their acquaintance. She reported that her feelings toward him were no longer those of fear or even sadness, but instead "like two old friends who have quarreled and don't quite know how to make up."

She was given the posthypnotic suggestion that she continue to work through her problem in the following form:

Of course, it will not be possible for you to keep Rover indefinitely. As you pointed out today, it would be so nice to have Rover really there. I think you can have Rover *really there* in a sense that down through the years

Rover has always been there in every dog that you met, particularly in little, frisky dogs. Each dog has been Rover as you looked at him with your little-girl eyes. If you work hard at becoming friends with Rover, your fear will leave you and you will quite naturally develop a greater acceptance of all dogs. As time goes on you will develop the idea of having a real Rover for you to enjoy and especially for Judy, who needs and wants a Rover of her own.

A relatively brief session was held one month later. The patient reported that five days after the previous session she had gone skating with her daughter and met several dogs. "It seemed very natural to reach down and pet them. There was no fear of doing it. They did not *feel* like dogs used to feel. I heard Judy yell, 'Oh, look, Mommy used to be afraid of dogs and isn't anymore,' and then it dawned on me that I really wasn't. It seemed that right after that I lost Rover." Laughingly she inquired, "You don't have him around here anymore, do you?" She stated that the family was now actively looking for a dog. She also presented the therapist with an unsolicited narration concerning her daily feelings and reactions during treatment. Three weeks later, the patient phoned to report that she had purchased a black Cocker Spaniel puppy and had named it "Happy Siesta," reflecting her reaction to the "hypnotic sleep" and a compromise of her desire to name it after me (Siesta = C. S., my first two initials).

Followup

Followups at one, five, and ten years have been undertaken. The patient has been symptom-free for 10 years now from a highly disruptive fear which preoccupied her for more than 40 years. Almost one year to the day later, the first followup interview was held with the patient. She began the session with the question, "Suppose the event I recalled wasn't true: could the mind make up something like that?" Discussion revealed other evidence of some residual resistance against a complete emotional acceptance of her childhood trauma; for instance, some elements of the experience were now incompletely remembered, and she described the memory as "not quite real." She also reported that while her mother continued to deny that the event had ever happened, a brother had confirmed the existence of a family dog named Rover and also the fact that she and her sister had been left momentarily alone at the time of the fatal accident because the two brothers, who had been carrying in wood, had gone to witness a fire at a neighbor's. Her younger sister also recalled that the patient had anxiously protected her in the presence of any and all dogs.

There was considerable circumstantial evidence to support the occurrence of a traumatic experience of the nature reported by the patient. Most convincing, possibly, is a congruence to the known dynamic structure basic to many phobic reactions; that is, the phobia dates from a fear-provoking episode in childhood, usually involving a severe disturbance in the parent-child relationship. Associated anxiety, shame, and guilt result in suppression and eventual repression of the frightening experience, leaving only the residual phobic symptom.

It was explained to the patient that it was relatively unimportant whether the memory of her childhood experience was correct in every detail, that the important factor was the effect of the therapeutic experience on her present adjustment. She reaffirmed that therapy had somewhat altered her relationship with her mother, daughter, and husband. The most evident effect of psychotherapy, however, continued to be a marked change in the patient's attitude toward dogs. "All of my life the touch of one gave me a feeling of something horrible. I'm still surprised that I feel so differently now."

In a letter at the fifth-year followup, she wrote:

> The fear of dogs has never returned. I still do not like to have dogs jump up on me, but I believe this is a normal reaction. It does not come from fear, but a desire to save hosiery and clothes. My daughter still has a dog, and I am certainly not afraid of him. I am not aware of any new fears that might have replaced the old one. In fact, I think I am generally less afraid of most things than are most people. I think I might be less inhibited than

most people. I used to be quite shy. This doesn't sound like a statement from a shy person, does it?

My wife and I happened to visit with my ex-patient and her family about a year later and during the process were introduced to her delightful teenage daughter's dog. We have exchanged two or three letters a year (as I do frequently with my former patients), and when I indicated to her about seven months ago that a publisher was interested in her personal story and possibly in reproducing some of the therapeutic interviews on tape, she immediately expressed her willingness and included the picture which faces p. 78 of this book.

Transcribed Excerpts from Therapy Sessions

Session IV, February 3

[This crucial session is included in its entirety. It is an excellent example of how a posthypnotic dream sheds light on the etiology of the patient's current problem.]

T: How did things go over the weekend?

P: Umm, fine. I kept my dreams. I did not dream Friday night, and Preston said he didn't think I slept much Saturday night to dream because Judy was ill; we were up and down all night with her, but apparently I did have one. Do you want to read them or do you want me to read them to you? You probably couldn't read my handwriting anyhow. Well, let's see, it was Saturday night when I had this one. It was about two little girls, toddler's size, and it was a very disturbing dream, incidentally. I woke up horribly frightened. One child was playing with the other as if she were a doll, and she was carrying her, putting her face next to hers, but the one that was being carried around was dead. But I went to sleep worrying about Judy so that might account for that, and it seems as if the live one was my little girl and I was distressed when she picked up the dead one because she did not realize it was dead. I was worried. I'm reading it just like I wrote it down. I asked the undertaker what sort of embalming fluid he used and if that would hurt my little girl. My concern seemed to be for Judy. Then there was something about redressing the dead baby and I was concerned about this. The undertaker or somebody was dressing it on a bed and I was very sad because it was lying so still. Then it seemed as if the dead one were mine and I was trying to get a box of a specific size, but I can't remember what the specific size was, to put things in them. I needed the big box to put the little boxes in. It seemed like I needed them for clothes or toys or something.

And then it seemed as if I were at my sewing machine, mending a badly torn dress. But then suddenly I realized that I wouldn't need it, that my child was dead and I cried a lot in the dream. Then it seemed there was only one child, the dead one, and it was mine. And I have written here that it was a very sad and disturbing dream.

And then Sunday night — did you say something?

T: No, just interested in your dream.

P: Well, I'm interested in that one. I never woke up from a dream like that. Horrible, oh, I would sorta recall it in the daytime, and almost shuddered. It was a terrible dream. And I didn't have anything to drink before I went to bed. And then Sunday night, it was rather vague, that's what I had written down first, but as I recorded it, it seemed to come back to me. It was something about wanting to get flowers to plant and Judy was with me, and we were visiting some friends on a hill, a pleasing grassy hill, and I left to go back to get some things in my car. I have the impression it was an old car, but not a car I had ever seen in my lifetime. Some people went back to the car with me and I expected Judy to follow, but she didn't. And I went back to find her but there was a crowd and I couldn't find her and I was quite angry with her for not coming with me. And while looking for her I saw some people using stones to build some sort of a formal garden, and it was pretty and I was interested in it. And they had lots of flowers and plants and they were bronze chrysanthemums. And I asked where they got so many flowers and they said a playground down the road was being torn up for a building site and there might be enough flowers so that I could get some to plant if I wanted them. They said they were making a formal garden and I was much amused at this. No, it looked like a formal garden to me and I asked them what they were doing and they said — no, I'm not reading this right. They *were* making a formal garden and I was amused because they said the filling station would be there. That's right, where they were making a formal garden and it looked funny because it didn't look like it was going to be a filling station, it looked like it would be a formal garden, and it didn't look like a place where one would put a filling station. And then I was very sorry that I had been angry with Judy for I realized she was little and probably could not find her way in the crowd. And I couldn't recall whether I ever found her or not, but I was awfully sorry when I woke up that I had been angry with her. That's all. Sorry about that mess-up, but I didn't have a chance to rewrite this, and I couldn't read what I had written.

T: Were you surprised to have these dreams and remember them?

P: No, because — I was surprised that that one was so horrible. It was a terrible dream. I wasn't surprised to remember them because you had told me to write them down and I had my cards and my pencil there.

T: You didn't have any trouble recalling them?

P: Well, at first I did. You see, it says "rather vague," but then as I started to record it would come to me. And one reason this one was hard to read as I finished it, there was something I remembered and I put in there, and that's why I was surprised to have such a horrible dream because I don't usually have; I don't usually remember my dreams in the first place, and I don't ever recall a horrible dream like that.

T: This business of digging up the past can be a little painful, can't it?

P: Yes, and oddly enough, a funny thing, when I woke from that horrible dream on Saturday night, when I awakened, before I even had a chance to write it down, yes, I think I recorded that because I was afraid I'd forget it, I recalled my little sister's death and I haven't thought of that for many, many, many years, because, gee, that happened — I recall practically nothing about it. One or two things but, oh, it's so long ago, I just never think about that.

T: How long ago was that?

P: Well, now let's see, if I tell you the whole truth I'll tell you my age, and a woman should never do that. But I'm not modest, so I will. Well, it was, it must have been about 41 years ago, I was about four or four and a half. I was too small to recall much about it and just two or three things that I remembered through the years. But that whole thing, I mean not the whole thing but just that, remembering that, and it shocked me that I would think of that after all these years.

T: Somehow this dream restimulated the memory?

P: Well, I don't know. I wonder, because I have not thought about that, oh, I'm sure I haven't for many, many years. But I thought of that and I thought it might be important and that's why I wrote it down; I was afraid I might forget. And there are only about two or three things that I remember about that incident, and one of them I seem to recall and that was one of the older ladies saying, "Let her go in there and see her if she wants to," or something like that. And that is something I remember, that I wanted to go in the room where she was. She was younger, she was about two, I guess, and I was about four. But I don't remember very much about it. Except one thing that has been interesting to me down through the years is how, the way children's minds can be, the things that adults say to them can be so misinterpreted. I guess the elderly ladies in the neighborhood, in trying to make me feel happier about it, had told me that my sister had gone away, and I guess they were trying to describe some sort of a heaven to me. But what they put in my mind was that she was way far away and way high up. Now that's all that was implanted there. And then the following year, my folks moved away from this little country town in southeast Missouri to St. Louis and I was quite happy; I can still remember that because I thought it was going far away. And I was even happier when we got to St. Louis because we got off at that Tower Grove station, and you know you have to go up a whole lot of stairs, and I thought, "Well, my little sister would be up there." But of course she wasn't and I thought, "Now, those ladies, they foxed me!" But that's been interesting to me as I've gotten older to realize that you must be very careful what you say to a child about things that are important; they don't understand.

But that's about all that I remember.

T: Do either of these dreams have any meaning to you?

P: No. I thought Judy seems to be definitely in one of them, and I presume since I thought the one child was mine, it was probably Judy, but they don't mean anything to me.

T: Well, would you like to explore into them and see what they might mean?

P: Well, yes, except I, this Saturday night one was so horrible, I kept hoping that I wouldn't have to go into that, it was sort of, it was so horrible that it sort of, well, I guess frightened me a little bit.

T: It frightened you that some harm might come to Judy?

P: No, oh, it was a horrible dream, I don't know why it seemed so horrible. No, no, I didn't really specifically connect her with the first dream.

T: Well, it's certainly up to you.

P: I know, and I think everybody feels sometimes that you want to and you don't want to. I want to get through this thing, 'cause when I clean house I clean out all the corners. You know, I really do, I want to get through with it. If it has something to do with it, why, I want to find out what.

T: Well, I think you can readily see that very often the things that people are most reluctant to look at or explore into or talk about are the very things which are causing their difficulties.

P: Yes, I know.

T: And so this thing which you describe as so horrible may in a sense be a key to your problem.

P: Yes, it may be. I don't know how or why. The only similarity to anything in my life is my sister's death, which I hadn't thought of in many years, but I don't remember anything connected with that that should upset me. I don't remember anything like that.

T: But it is odd that that should come about.

P: Yes, it is odd that I should have thought about that in such a sort of a fearful way. When I awakened, I felt fearful. I rather expect to find my two "ornery" brothers siccing their dogs on me, that's what I expect to find. Maybe I won't find that.

T: Well, if you think you can stand up to this. . . .

P: I can stand up to anything.

T: All right.

P: I hope.

T: Well, let's find out, shall we?

P: I guess so.

T: This may be rather painful to you, as you realize, but I have confidence in the fact that apparently you're the type of person who can bear quite a bit of pain and anxiety and had to in the past. And there is always the fact, of course, that this is something that happened to you over 40 years ago.

P: Uh-huh.

T: And what you're really doing is reacting to this as you did probably as a little girl.

P: Uh-huh.

T: And what we want here, this is in a sense what we were talking about the other day in connection with this dog, that the grown-up part of you recognizes that there is nothing to be afraid of a little friendly puppy.

P: Uh-huh.

T: But there, too, you react as if you were a little girl, don't you?

P: Yes, and I *am* afraid. Saturday when we were out with the sled and the horses, there were dogs yapping around the horses, and I was obviously afraid. Preston laughed and told the puppy to come back next week and I'd be friendlier then. But I was afraid. And then we walked to class the other morning and we met five or six dogs and I thought, "Now which of those dogs am I the most afraid of?" And I wasn't afraid of the great big ones, it was that little old pesky one that was jumping around. And I wasn't afraid it would bite me; I don't know what I'm afraid of. I act just like a child, I guess you'd say, when they come around. No adult should act that way. I can't help it, I'm afraid.

T: But you still have a child's feelings.

P: I surely do, and I'm afraid.

T: Then perhaps the answer to this does lie someplace way back in childhood.

P: It must, because as long as I can remember, I've been afraid. And you would laugh to know how many dinner invitations I have turned down because I knew somebody had a dog in the house. Now that's as abnormal as it can be, isn't it? Don't answer. I know it is.

T: Well, there are actually a lot of people who have something specific like that that they are afraid of.

P: Well, yes, the only encouraging thing is when this Dr. Jones said he has yet to meet a normal person. I know it's abnormal and I'd like very much to be rid of it.

T: Well, we'll see if you feel it is worth the price.

P: Oh, I think it would be worth most anything, I really do, I really do.

T: Then let's show me by how deeply you go under today, because you will probably have to go rather deeply to face up to this. You ready?

P: I'm ready.

[Hypnosis is induced by the tapping method.]

T: Now, I told you when we met last Friday that you would have a dream or dreams related to this fear that you have of dogs. And you complied very nicely; you brought in two dreams, even though the first of them made you very anxious. You nevertheless demonstrated the fact, I think, right there that you were going to face up to this thing, even though you found it temporarily painful. You had, of course, already demonstrated in the other session your ability to face up to painful past experiences. Now we have one more to go, one more to go, with the possibility that when you have recovered this memory and talked about it and thought about it and lived it, and lived with it for a little while, that you will finally, after all these years, be able to establish control of this pesky fear that has bothered you.

Now, I'm very interested in this dream that you had Saturday night. And I think we should look at it closely and carefully. Now you seem to have done a faithful job of recording it, but I think, in order to assure ourselves you haven't forgotten any important details, that you should experience this dream again. But as you pointed out, it was intensely painful to you at the time, so I'm going to try to help you to remove yourself somewhat from the dream, so that rather than have you actually re-experience the dream as you could if I suggested this, I want you to go back to the movie theater, back to the theater; remember the movie theater you were in last time? And I want you to seat yourself there in the movie theater. You can see it, it's the one you were in there at the hospital, it's a small theater. Only you and I are there now. We're there together. You must never forget that I am there beside you. In front of you is the blank screen. In a moment I am going to snap my fingers. When

I do, you will see a movie of the dream you had, a movie of the dream you had on Saturday night. You will see it just as it happened, in every detail. You will see it in every detail, just as it occurred. When the movie begins, I want you to lift your index finger on the left hand; when it is completed, I want you to lower your finger. Then I want you to tell me about it, exactly as you saw it on the screen. Do you understand?

P: Yes.

T: All right, the projectionist is getting ready. He is mounting the movie on the camera, putting the reel on. In a moment you will see a movie as clearly and vividly as you dreamt it, in all its detail. However, it will be less disturbing to you because you will continue to remember that you are actually seated here in the movie theater. You are seated here in the movie theater, only *looking* at the screen. Do you understand that?

P: Yes.

T: All right. Now looking ahead at the screen, you can see it there clearly, it's a white screen, you're looking at it, he is putting on the reel, snapping the button, and here comes the picture. [Pause.] Watch the screen, watch it closely. As the movie begins, I want you to indicate it by raising the index finger of your left hand. Can you see the screen?

P: Yes.

T: Can you see a movie on it?

P: No.

T: All right, now what do you think happened there?

P: I'm afraid.

T: I know you're afraid. Can you face this or not?

P: Yes, I want to.

T: It's up to you whether he runs the movie or not.

P: I know.

T: If you're too afraid . . .

P: No, I want to.

T: All right, then here we go again. You're sitting there in the movie theater, I'm seated there beside you. In a moment, if you are able to face it, and really want to find out, the movie will begin. When it does begin, I want you to signal this to me by raising the index finger of your left hand, letting it fall when the movie is over. You will remember at all times that you are seated there in the movie theater, and that I am there to help you. When you are ready, he will begin the film. When you are ready, when you can face it. There is the screen, look at it closely. Now, when you are ready.

You will remember it just as you experienced it, in all of its detail, except that you will remember that you are outside of it, just sitting there watching it; watch carefully everything that happens.

[After a 30-second lapse, the patient signals that the "movie" has begun. The patient looks obviously preoccupied and somewhat disturbed. Five minutes and 10 seconds elapse.]

T: Is the movie over now?

P: I don't think so.

T: All right, go on. See the rest of it. [Pause.] Is there still something there?

P: Yes.

T: Go on, take your time. See it all, clearly, vividly, completely. [Pause.] Is it through now?

P: No.

T: Can you see it clearly?

P: Not too clearly.

T: All right, tell me as much as you can about what is happening, what you saw there on the screen.

P: There was a room. There are two children. One is carrying the other and then my mother came. It doesn't look like my mother, but it's my mother and she told me to put the baby down and I did. And then my mother and my father seem to be tired or ill or something. They're in the bed in the next room. And someone is changing the clothes and I found the big box that I couldn't find before [in the nocturnal dream] and they put the baby in the box on the bed. And my mother told me I should not touch the box. I can look but I cannot touch the box. And so I don't want to touch the box. Then it is kind of hazy and that is all I know.

T: What is it, do you think, that you have been telling me here?

P: I guess it happened to me. And there is that dress, it was torn.

T: Whose dress was it?

P: It was the baby's dress and it was torn.

T: How did it get torn?

P: I don't know how it got torn. It got torn. I don't know whether I tore it or somebody else tore it.

T: Where did you see the dress?

P: The dress, after it was torn? After it wasn't on the baby. I don't know.

T: All right, now listen to me. Is there more of this?

P: Well, there seems to be a little black dog but I don't know for sure that there is. But if there is, I'm not afraid of it. I don't know but there seems to be.

T: A little black dog?

P: Yes, with curly black hair, but I am not afraid of it because it's in that room too, and I don't feel afraid of it.

T: Uh-huh. Now, I want you to listen carefully to me. You know fortune tellers and people like that employ crystal balls and they claim they can see the future in it. I'm not at all sure about that, but I do know that in looking into a crystal ball, you often find it easy to see things in yourself, to see forgotten experiences and memories. I want you now to look in the crystal ball. You're in a room, in a room, and it's completely dark, draped on all sides, except there on the table in the middle of the room is a luminous crystal ball. Can you see it?

P: I can see it.

T: All right. There is a crystal ball, you can see it very clearly, very clearly. I want you to go over, sit down, and stare into the crystal ball, stare into the crystal ball, stare at it intensely, and as you stare, as you stare, added details of the things you've been telling me about will appear. Added details, pictures of the past, pictures concerned with what was happening there in that room. Pictures concerned with your little sister, you and your relationship to her, and also the little black dog. Stare at it, and as you stare, simply tell me the things that appear to you. Tell me the picture that you see there. Describe them to me.

P: My Aunt Ethel is standing there. [Moans.] My little sister and I are playing.

T: Turn your head this way so I can hear you more clearly. Go on.

P: My little sister and I are playing. And there is a little dog there. My little sister is a pretty little girl. And there is a woodpile, a piece of wood, some wood. [Moans.] My brothers are there too.

T: Uh-huh.

P: They are carrying wood. My little sister has some pieces of wood in her hands, in her arms. I don't have any.

T: Go on; as you continue to look into the crystal ball, more and more pictures continue to flood their way.

P: There is that same little dog.

T: Whose little dog is it?

P: I don't know but it is staying with me.

T: It must have a name of some sort. All little dogs have a name.

P: I don't know it.

T: Now listen carefully; perhaps you can hear somebody call it by name. [Claps.]

P: My mother is at the door; she is calling the little dog "Rover."

T: What is she calling it?

P: Rover.

T: Rover?

P: It's going.

T: That must be its name then.

P: [Moans.] That's its name. It knocked my little sister over.

T: Oh?

P: She fell on the wood.

T: Your little sister fell on the wood?

P: The wood she had in her hands. She's all right.

T: It didn't really hurt her very much?

P: I guess not.

T: Go on.

P: Mother took her in the house, then I went in the house, and we are in the house now.

T: Tell me about the house and what is going on.

P: Mother is looking at her face. Velma, that's her name. It's bleeding — on the cheek.

T: She got a scratch on the cheek?

P: She has a scratch. [Pause.] That seems to be all.

T: All right. Now as you continue to look into the crystal ball, staring at it intently, you'll find still other pictures, pictures relating to your life there in the family, the tragedy of your little sister's death, and the little black dog. Stare at it, look into it, and way, way down in the depth you can see pictures forming, and they seem to grow in size and float up to the top. What do you see now?

P: Well, there is a door from the room that leads onto the porch, the back porch. My mother thinks I knocked my sister over.

T: Your mother thinks you knocked your little sister over?

P: And so they are going to play a little game. My brothers, my big sister, and I are going to walk to the door, and when the one gets to the door who knocked my sister over, something will knock on the other side. And when I get to the door, something knocks, but I didn't knock her over.

T: What happens now?

P: Well, when I go to the door, something knocks on the other side, but I didn't knock her over, but everybody thinks I did, and they don't believe me when I tell them. But I wouldn't hurt her.

T: Was it there in the yard when they thought you knocked her over?

P: Yes, when she was running with the wood.

T: Actually, it was the little dog.

P: The dog was playing with her.

T: And you got blamed for it?

P: I was just watching it.

T: You got blamed for it?

P: I got blamed for it. I didn't do it.

T: Go on, tell me what happens next.

P: We're back in the living room, and they think I did it, but I didn't knock her over. And that's all there is.

T: There's more to this. What did they do to you? Look in the crystal ball — what did they do to you because of that?

P: I guess my mother's spanking me.

T: She's spanking you?

P: I guess so.

T: How did she do it? Describe it.

P: I am on her lap and she's spanking me. Everybody's watching. I don't like it.

T: How do you feel?

P: I don't like it because I didn't do it. I wouldn't mind being spanked if I did it, but I didn't do it.

T: So you are being punished for something you didn't do?

P: That's it.

T: Go on.

P: I'm in bed now, I'm in my own bed now.

T: What are you thinking there in your bed?

P: I wish they knew I didn't do it.

T: You feel badly?

P: [Sadly] I am unhappy.

T: Just keep talking about this and what happens next. As you look there in the ball, the scenes, the old feelings, the memories, the smells, everything comes alive almost as if it were happening now.

P: My big sister's there, because I sleep in her bed. She is comforting me. I think she doesn't think I did it. I don't think she thinks I did it. She was always my friend. And now it's morning, I guess. Seems sort of cold in the house. It's breakfast time but I'm not going to eat because I don't feel good. They blame me. I am unhappy about it.

Seems like I'm in the yard again, and the dog is there in the yard with me.

T: Is this the next day?

P: Yes, this is the next day.

T: All right, come on.

P: And we're out by the woodpile again and I feel quite badly because they think I pushed my sister over and I didn't, and my little sister isn't out playing with me. She is ill. She's ill, I guess, and Dr. Donahue is coming. That's Dr. Donahue coming. Then there are a lot of people there. My mother seems to be crying and my dad too. My little sister just looks like she's asleep.

T: Your little sister?

P: My little sister, she just looks like she is asleep. She is awfully pretty.

T: Where is she?

P: She is lying on a bed. No, it isn't a bed, it looks like an ironing board. Oh, I'm looking for something and I am finding it now. It is a necklace. It is mine and I ask my Aunt Ethel to put it on her because it will look pretty on her, and my Aunt Ethel does. She looks awfully pretty. Now everybody is in the parlor, it seems as if they are, and that's Gordon coming in.

T: Everyone is in the parlor?

P: Yes, everybody's in the parlor now, and when Gordon comes in, they all start crying again.

T: Who's Gordon?

P: He was my sister's husband, but they were not married then. Velma always liked him. And he goes in and sees her, she's awfully pretty, and I go too. Then we come back out in the parlor and he's holding my hand because he likes us both. Then I go back in by myself. I want to see her again. She looks so pretty lying there, so I think I'll pick her up. She doesn't hug me like she usually does, though. I am holding her and the dog is with me. He wants to see her too. Oh, he tore her dress!

T: Pardon?

P: He tore her dress.

T: How did he do that?

P: He was jumping up on her, just playing, and he tore her dress. Oh, Mother will die.

T: Pardon?

P: My mother won't like that!

T: She won't like it because the dog . . .

P: Oh, no, the dog shouldn't be in the house, but I don't think I let him in. I know I should put her down, but I want to hold her. I know I shouldn't but I want to hold her.

T: What do you think and feel about her?

P: Oh, she's so pretty and sweet. And I just want to hold her.

T: What happens next?

P: My mother came into the room. She's mad at me. She told me I should know better. Somebody took the baby away from me.

T: You didn't want to give her up?

P: No, I wanted to hold her. It must be my Aunt Anna. She said I shouldn't have torn her dress. Oh, but I didn't tear her dress. I didn't do it.

T: [Simulating the mother.] Somebody did! It's torn!

P: I didn't do it.

T: Well, who did it?

P: Rover did it, but he didn't mean to.

T: Rover tore the dress?

P: Rover tore the dress, but he didn't mean to. He just wanted to see her. Why doesn't that place on her face go away?

T: She still has the scratch?

P: Oh, yes. It looks like a splinter in it. But Aunt Anna, she'll fix it, she'll change her dress and it'll be all right. And she'll put the necklace back on her, and now it's all right.

T: She's got a new dress and the necklace on her?

P: Yes, she's got a new dress and necklace and a bracelet on her arm. I think that it's mine too. Yes, I want her to have it. Now they are going to put her in that box. I mustn't touch the box, but I can look over her if somebody is with me.

I guess we are going somewhere now. Oh, yes, we are going [pause — sighs very deeply].

T: Going where?

P: Going behind Aunt Ethel's house to the cemetery. They are putting the box down in the ground. We are singing some kind of songs. I wish I could see her again, but I guess I won't.

T: Your little sister is gone now?

P: Uh-huh. It seems like it's later, some days later. I am on the back porch by myself. I wish she would come play with me.

T: You're lonely now?

P: Mother comes out the back door and she finds me crying. I don't want her to find me crying.

T: You don't want her to know how you feel?

P: No, she thinks I hurt her and I didn't.

T: Your mother blames you for what happened to your little sister?

P: She thinks I pushed her over. But I didn't. [Pause.] I don't seem to like my dog anymore.

T: He still wants to be friendly, doesn't he?

P: I don't want him to be friendly.

T: You don't like your little dog?

P: No, I don't like my little dog anymore. I want my sister. I don't want that little old dog.

T: Your little dog took your sister away from you?

P: I don't like him. I wish that they would take *him* away.

T: You want him to go away and your little sister to come back?

P: Yes.

T: Go on.

P: I am just lonely.

T: You're terribly lonely after your sister is gone?

P: Yes.

T: And unhappy because your mother blames you? You don't like your dog anymore?

P: No.

T: This feeling must go on for quite a while, doesn't it?

P: I guess so.

T: All right. Now look into the ball again, look into the crystal ball. Other thoughts and feelings are coming to mind about what happened to you then. Later thoughts and feelings — your feelings about your sister, your feelings about your mother, your mother's feelings about you, and your feelings about Rover.

P: I wish she would give me to my Aunt Ethel.

T: You want to give the dog away?

P: No, I wish my mother had given me to my Aunt Ethel. She nearly did.

T: You were so unhappy you wanted to be away from your mother?

P: I guess so. She nearly gave me to her when I was born, because she nearly died and they said she should give me to somebody. She gave me to my Aunt Ethel but she lived. Now I wish my Aunt Ethel had me.

T: Why?

P: She doesn't blame me. She knows I wouldn't do that.

T: How does your mother keep reminding you?

P: [Sighs.] When I tell her I miss Velma, she says it is my fault. It is not my fault.

T: When you tell her how you miss your little sister, she says it is your fault she is gone?

P: It is not my fault!

T: How does it make you feel?

P: I am *so* unhappy. She should see it is not my fault; Rover pushed her over.

T: Didn't you tell her this?

P: She doesn't believe me. Nobody believes me.

T: Nobody believes you?

P: Maybe my big sister does. I guess *she* does, but my mother doesn't.
T: How about your father?
P: I don't know about Dad.
T: Your brothers?
P: I don't know about them.
T: It is mainly your mother, then, who blames you? She makes you feel very unhappy.
P: She is lonely, too, though.
T: And how do you feel during this time about Rover?
P: I don't much want to play with him anymore.
T: Why not? What do you feel about him?
P: I don't like him anymore.
T: Why?
P: Well, he pushed her over. He tore her dress, I didn't.
T: He pushed her over, he tore your dress?
P: He didn't tear *my* dress, he tore *her* dress.
T: And besides that he got your mother angry at you? So he is to blame for all this and yet *you're* the one who gets punished.
P: I wish they would take him to my grandfather's farm.
T: You want him to go away so you won't have to see him anymore. Does he remind you of what happened?
P: Yes.
T: What finally happens to Rover?
P: I guess he goes to Grandfather's farm.
T: So they do send him away. And what happens to you?
P: I have to stay there.

T: You can't go away?

P: I wish I could go to Aunt Ethel's.

T: You would be happier away from your mother?

P: Uh-huh.

T: Any other pictures come to mind?

P: It seems as if I have some flowers in my hand and I am going up back of Aunt Ethel's house. I have to hurry because if Mother catches me she won't like it. But Aunt Ethel sees me. She goes with me and that is better. She helps me plant them. Then we come back down the hill together in the lane there. I tell her good-bye, but she thinks she had better go with me and she takes me home.

T: Does she tell your mother where you have been?

P: No.

T: Aunt Ethel sort of understands a little more, doesn't she?

Now listen to me. You had another dream. It was rather vague, something about flowers, Judy being with you, and about losing Judy in the crowd, and you saw people building a formal garden with stones and lots of flowers, and you were amused because they said there would be a filling station there. Later you found Judy and you were sorry that you had been angry with her because she was so little.

P: I don't know if I found her.

T: You don't know, but you were sorry you had been angry with her?

P: Oh, yes.

T: All right. Now this dream which you had, this dream that you told me about — look into the ball, look into the crystal ball, can you see it there clearly? What is the relation of this dream to what you have been telling me? There is a relationship, a very definite one. Look into the crystal ball and as you do so, the dream will be transformed and like pieces of a jigsaw puzzle, will come out, piece by piece, so that you'll understand what the dream meant in relation to what you have been talking about. The pictures are beginning to form. At first they're far away. Now they're becoming clearer and clearer, bigger and bigger. And there's a picture. Describe to me the pictures as they appear.

P: They seem like a — like a — like Laurel Hill Cemetery in St. Louis.

T: Uh-huh.

P: That's the, there are men down there, they're building some pretty fences. Well, it seems — that is funny.

T: Just tell me as the pictures appear, describe them to me.

P: It seems as if there are lots of people going up there. I guess that is my older sister's death. Yes, that is my older sister. They are burying her there in that cemetery.

T: Other pictures are appearing one after the other, pushing their way up clearly, so that you can understand piece by piece what your dreams meant to you.

P: Oh, the filling station. [Sighs.] That is when we were coming from Carbondale to St. Louis in the funeral procession. We stopped so the cars could get some gas. My brother-in-law got a Coke. It seemed odd, that he'd want a Coke. I guess he didn't even think. [Pause.] We are back in the cemetery. They are burying my sister.

T: In the dream that you had, you dreamt that Judy became separated from you and you could not find her there in the crowd and you were very sorry you had become angry with her. What does that mean to you now?

P: I don't know.

T: Look there in the crystal ball, look into the crystal ball. There are other pictures forming which will tell you the meaning of that part of your dream. Pushing their way up, becoming clearer and clearer. Describe to me what you see now.

P: My sister-in-law, she said I should have come down for the operation instead of her; but I was going to go take care of my sister. I would have gone but we didn't expect her to die. I was going to go take care of her.

T: Your sister-in-law implied you had neglected her?

P: She thought I should have been down there for the operation.

T: You had no way of knowing she was going to die?

P: No, I was going to take care of her.

T: You must have felt badly, of course, when she did and you didn't see her.

T: I saw her.

T: Oh, before she died?

P: I saw her die.

T: Oh, you did see her die?

P: But I wasn't there for the operation.

T: I see. Well, what does it mean, then, when you say you are sorry you had been angry with Judy?

P: I don't know, because I wasn't angry with anybody that I know of.

T: Because she was little and couldn't find her way in the crowd?

P: I don't know. Judy wasn't there. I don't understand it.

T: All right now, listen to my voice and what I'm saying. Listen to me. In a moment I'm going to snap my fingers. When I do, you're going to have a second dream, another dream, which will mean the same as the first dream, the dream you had Sunday night. It will mean the same, but it will be clearer to you, less confused, and you will better be able to understand what it means. The dream is beginning to form now, beginning to form; in a moment the dream will occur. A dream which means the same as the other dream, but which may be a little more direct, clearer to you, and less confused. Now it's going to start and when it starts, I want you to raise your index finger and when it stops I want you to lower your finger. It's beginning now, ready to start [snaps fingers], the dream is ready to go. It's forming, pushing its way up, pushing up. Are you ready for it now?

P: It's not clear.

T: Tell me about it.

P: I don't know.

T: All right, now listen to what I'm saying. It's important that you face this. There are apparently other feelings here. There are apparently other feelings here. Are you ready now?

P: Yes.

T: All right. Tell me what you've been thinking about.

P: I've been thinking about the dream.

T: Tell me what you thought about it, will you please?

P: I was thinking about, what does it mean?

T: And what came to mind?

P: I don't know, I can't understand it; I mean, I don't know what.

T: It's still confused?

P: It's confusing.

T: All right, now listen to what I have to say here, if you will please. And that is that our time is almost up for this afternoon. I think rather than having you dream again now, I would prefer, if it's all right with you, if we follow the same procedure we did over the weekend. And that is, I'll plan to see you again in a few days and in the meantime, I want you to again pay close attention to your dreams. And you will find that again you will have one or more dreams which are related, which are closely related to your concern, your fear about dogs. I think we have made considerable progress this afternoon in understanding your fear of little dogs, don't you?

P: I think so.

T: I think so too. There may be more, however, and if there is, we should know that. But you will find that as you recover these memories, that your concern about dogs will naturally be decreased. I think it is very easy to see how you could have these intense feelings about dogs from what you've told me thus far.

But between now and when we meet again, and now I am talking to the very deepest recesses of your unconscious, I want you to have one or more dreams which you will clearly experience and remember about your concern about dogs. I think you can see that what you thought was a fairly specific fear, and probably went back to a single specific instance, was actually closely involved and woven into a great many things, thoughts, feelings that happened to you as a little girl.

As I said, I think we have made good progress in a short time. In another session or two we should have a very clear understanding of how this fear arose and how it grew. So between now and the next session, as I said, I want you to have one or more dreams which will continue to provide us with information on how you developed this intense fear about dogs. I want you to have also another dream, a second dream which means the same as the first, the same as you had there on Sunday night, the vague one about the flowers and about losing Judy there, etc. I want you to have another dream which means the same but whose meaning will be clearer. Do you understand that?

P: Yes.

T: All right, now I want you to relax. Are there any other questions or any other points or anything that you want to bring up at this time that you think may be of importance here?

P: I don't think so.

T: Do you think we have covered everything you want to talk about now?

P: I don't think of anything else.

T: All right. Now I want you to go very deeply asleep in a moment, so that when I awaken you it will be as from a very deep sleep. You will remember as much of what we have talked about as you can face. As much of what we have talked about as you can face. I am going to leave it up to you. Your mind will protect you in the same way that it has been protecting you all these years. You can so readily see the way the mind has of locking away painful thoughts, memories, feelings. Go deeply asleep. Very deeply asleep. Now I want you to sleep deeply for a couple of minutes, and I will awaken you.

[Instructions preparatory to awakening:] We've talked about your little sister's death and how distressing it was to you. And from the way in which you describe it, the way in which it came about and the fact that you were blamed for it certainly must have been a disturbing thing to you. It would be, of course, to any child. But, nevertheless, you are facing it perhaps as you have not faced it since you've grown up and become an adult, and as an adult, you can face it, painful as it is, knowing that it was something that happened to you many, many years ago.

And it was something for which you were not to blame. Something for which you could not blame yourself. Now through the next few days until we meet again, unconsciously all the pieces will begin to fall in place, the pieces of this jigsaw puzzle, the most evident symptom of which was your fear of dogs. You will come to an unconscious understanding of your concern about death and your relationship to death — what it meant to you when your little sister died, what it meant to you when your bigger sister died, what it meant when your two babies died. How all of this falls into a pattern. As I said, these pieces will assemble themselves unconsciously. I don't want you to let it come too close to the surface yet, not until we meet next time when I will be there to help you to face it, to assemble it. Then all the pieces, all of the material, the content that we have been stirring up the last couple of weeks, will begin to well up, to fall into place, and you will be able to remember, to experience, and talk about it. As I said, I don't want this to occur until you come back the next time. Instead, your unconscious will simply prepare you for all of this. Will prepare you to face this material, and when it is faced, you will recognize that your fear of dogs is only a symptom of something else, something that you feared more. You will be able to see this relationship clearly and as a result lose this concern about dogs, recognizing that it is no more the real problem than, say, the spots when a child has measles.

So that is your homework, and the next time, if you are ready, we will face all of these things, bring them out and talk about them and put everything as it should be so that you will no longer be as troubled as you have been the last few weeks, so that you will no longer have your phobia about dogs.

I think we've made good progress. I think you've been a very good patient, and certainly it has been painful but I think you've shown real courage in facing up to this material.

Now as I said, I am going to awaken you. You will awaken as if from a deep sleep. You will remember as much as you can face at the present time.

[Awakens patient.] That was a very deep and long sleep this time, wasn't it?

P: [Stretches.] This is better than I have slept the last two nights. [Looks off into space reflectively.]

T: What are you thinking about?

P: I was thinking Mother should have been angry with me.

T: Should she?

P: Well, I mean, I shouldn't have picked up the baby but I didn't know. I should not have done that, should I? It must have shocked her horribly.

T: You can understand how your mother must have felt?

P: Oh, yes.

T: Even though you also realize that as a little girl you couldn't have known?

P: Oh, no. Nobody ever mentioned that to me. I didn't know I did that.

T: That you had picked her up?

P: Uh-huh. I never knew that.

T: You can't quite say that you never knew it.

P: Well, I mean that I didn't remember it. In my conscious life I didn't know it had happened.

T: It's interesting, isn't it, how all of these details of our lives are stored away. Did you remember that the dog had jumped up?

P: Oh, no. I didn't remember ever having a dog.

T: Do you remember now?

P: Yes.

T: What was his name?

P: Rover. Perhaps he is the little rascal in that picture that they were holding. [In the first session she remarked that there was a photograph taken of herself at a very young age in which she was seated next to a dog held by her two brothers.] Isn't that funny, I don't remember ever having a dog.

T: But you do remember now?

P: Well, I guess so, it seems to be there.

T: How sure are you that you had this dog?

P: I can't prove it but I don't know, it just seems so.

T: In other words, the feeling is real.

P: I guess Mother could tell me.

T: Your mother is still alive?

P: My mother is still alive.

T: It would be interesting to check some of this with her.

P: I would like to know.

T: I think you should do that.

P: I would like to. My mother is an invalid in St. Louis. She lived with us after Dad's death for about a year and a half, but it didn't work out. She seemed to resent Judy. And so we didn't realize that was building up and the kindergarten teacher noticed that it seemed to be causing Judy some difficulty so we had to change that arrangement. I will just have to go to St. Louis and see her. She could tell me a lot of these things. I guess she would, unless it it was so horrible to her she wouldn't want to talk about it, but surely she could now, 'cause there is no one else. My Aunt Ethel isn't living and my sister isn't living. If my dad were living I could talk to him. I could talk to him about anything.

T: Your brothers?

P: Well, the one brother I could talk to best is in California. I don't see him very often. The other is in St. Louis and we have never been very close.

T: Do you ever remember that your mother had blamed you in this fashion?

P: Oh, no, oh, no, no. I didn't know Mother had blamed me. I can understand, though, some of my actions as a child now. I always wanted to please everybody, looking back over it from an adult point of view. And I can remember that at school I would take blame for things that other kids did and my mother would get real provoked with me because as a child, every, almost every week, she had to go to the principal. I guess I was a problem child. If the teacher wanted to blame somebody, I was always glad to take the blame. If anything were done and the teacher wanted to blame somebody, I was just real happy to say I did it. That was certainly an abnormality. As I grew older I realized it was just real stupid, but I think I didn't want to be blamed for anything. I mean I didn't want anybody to be blamed, so I would take the blame, that was it. It was mixed up, I know that. But I was always in some real difficulties. And I wanted people to like me as a child, I can remember. I expect that Mother must have been terribly upset about me picking up the baby. Of course, if she believed I had caused her to fall, of course, she would have blame me. I mean, it must have been awful for her.

T: Do you remember consciously, or did you remember your little sister's death?

P: I remember very little about it. I remember that she died.

T: Did you know of what?

P: I heard them talk about the doctor in this little town didn't seem to know what was the matter. And after she died, they removed a splinter from her face, and he thought perhaps it was an infection, and I heard them talk about that. But I didn't know what had happened, or anything about it.

T: Do you think your mother would admit to you that she had blamed you?

P: I doubt it.

T: It might be a very sensitive point with her.

P: I think it would be. I wouldn't want to ask her *that*, but I would like to know if she remembers these details that I didn't know anything about. It is rather hopeless, she wouldn't know if the dog pushed Velma down because I guess sincerely she thought I did.

T: Or at least that's the way you felt?

P: Uh-huh.

T: But she would probably remember the incident in the yard.

P: She surely would. She surely would. Anything as important as that.

T: Well, unless she did the same as you have done, that is, lock this away. Of course, you were a little girl, but even adults can do things like that about situations that are painful.

P: Do you think she would remember my picking up the baby?

T: Or the torn dress?

P: Yes, that must have horrified her. I know it did because when I had this dream, I shuddered, I mean to think that Judy would do something like that, or my child, I mean it must have been a horrible thing.

T: It's interesting. You put yourself in your mother's place in the dream, didn't you?

P: I guess I did, didn't I? I wonder why?

T: So that it was Judy instead of you.

P: Yes, and I was concerned about Judy's doing it, because . . . and yet it didn't really seem to be Judy in that first dream. It was just two children. The one that did the picking up seemed to be mine but was actually me instead of mine. If I had realized that yesterday, I would have shuddered, wouldn't I? It doesn't seem as bad now as it did yesterday. It just seems like an incident that must have been very shocking to my mother. I would like to know if she would remember any of these things.

T: There are a lot of details that you recalled here that you might mention to her.

P: Yes. It is funny I should have thought about my older sister's death. I don't know why. That wouldn't be connected with it in any way, would it?

T: I don't know.

P: Well, I had this fear so much longer ago than that. I don't see why it would be.

T: Let's let your unconscious work on that for a little while, shall we?

P: Well, I guess so.

T: You'll notice that through all of the sessions runs a theme about death.

P: Yes, I had noticed that and oddly enough, I don't think I feel, well, badly or unkindly of death. It is something I have thought a lot about and talked to a lot of people. Oh, for instance, a very good doctor-friend of ours, I had a chance once, we talked about it for a long while. I think the turning point of my thinking about death, if one has a turning point . . . well, let's say I thought about it differently after my older sister's death. If I had been afraid of it before, I wasn't afraid of it anymore, because she was, I guess, the best person I ever knew in my life, or one of the best. She was a very good person, she was a minister's wife and did more for everybody than most anybody else I've ever known. Her death really seemed unnecessary. She was only 39. But I saw her die. Seeing her die, it seemed to make me feel differently about death. It seemed like sorta, not a mysterious thing, something you might feel curious about, but not to fear. I have been thankful that I was there to see her die, if she had to die, because it gave me a different view about it.

T: Well, maybe you are already beginning to answer some of the questions of the relationship between the first experience and the second. As I said, let's leave that go for a little while. When do you want to meet again? I think one or two more sessions may be sufficient.

Session V, February 6

[This very short excerpt from the beginning of Session V is included because it reflects the changes in attitude that are already occurring in the thinking of the patient. She was beginning to alter her perspective of the meaning of "dogs" since she had relived the experience from childhood and has had the opportunity to view it from her adult point of view. The patient has definitely passed the "crisis point" in her treatment; never again would she be so totally sad and depressed.]

P: If there is any question about our making progress, we are. Tuesday morning when I went to class I wished I would meet a dog. I was curious as to how I would react. It must have been the first morning in weeks that I didn't meet a dog. But in coming back from class I met a big Collie. I thought, "I am going to pet him." And I felt differently towards a dog than I have ever felt. Is it possible to feel sorry for a dog? That is the way I felt. I was able to stroke his fur and pet him. I was doing real well until the Smith's dog saw what was happening. I guess he was so amazed at seeing me pet one of his friends that he decided that he would run over too. When I saw him coming I started saying, "Go away, go away." The same old thing. But I think we have made progress. I think that is the first time I ever willingly petted a dog. . . .

Session VI, February 10

[The following excerpt from Session VI constitutes only the final one-sixth of the session. It contains the suggestion for a hallucinated fantasy of the little dog which terrorized the patient as a small girl. The "dog" is a symbol of the disturbed relationship between the patient as a child and her mother.]

T: I want you to relax and let yourself go and I want these memories to fade and to dim, and go very deeply asleep, very deeply asleep. We are going to do something next which requires a very deep level of sleep, even deeper than you have ever gone before. Do you understand?

P: Yes.

T: In order to accomplish this you are going to have to go very deep, twice as deep as you ever allowed yourself to go before. Now let's begin far down the steps. What step would you say you are at, what level?

P: Thirty-five comes to my mind.

T: Now I want you to go down at least another 10 steps. With each step you will go very, very deeply. [The count is made to 45.] I am going. . . . [The therapist is interrupted by a phone call.]

In a moment I am going to awaken you, just as when you were in the dental office and saw the crystal ball — after you are seemingly awake and we are talking, I want you to gaze over in the corner underneath the washstand, and as you look over there, you will see a little puppy, a real dog, a little black dog. You will see him very clearly and very distinctly. He will be a friendly little puppy, and he will be quite interested in you and you quite interested in him. It will be clear, vivid to you, as clear and distinct and vivid as any dog you have ever seen. And perhaps you'll recognize him, perhaps not; I don't know whether you will. Remember after I awaken you and as we're talking, you look over to the corner and see this little, friendly black puppy dog. He will be very interested in you and you in him. Relax! Relax! In a moment I am going to awaken you. I do not want you to remember this suggestion after you awaken. I want you to forget about it, not try to think about it, not be consciously aware of it, although, of course, your unconscious will have complete awareness of what I have told you and will act on it.

[Patient is awakened.] Did you go very deeply today?

P: I must have been asleep pretty deep. When one's asleep in this chair, one doesn't snore, does one?

T: [Humorously] If they do, I wake them up usually.

P: Oh, good, is that why you woke me up now?

T: Actually you've been under quite some time — it's five o'clock already.

P: Is it really?

T: Time flies. How do you feel about things now?

P: Well, I guess, oh, just wishing I could make faster progress.

T: Well, I think you have done very well in this time, don't you?

P: Well, I guess so, yes, really, it's just that I'm an eager beaver. I want to get anything that I do done, wrapped up, and to get onto something else, I guess.

T: It takes a great deal of unlearning, though, don't you think—something which has existed so long?

P: Yes. [Patient stares intently into a corner of the office. Long pause.]

T: What are you looking at?

P: The corner of your room.

T: What's there?

P: Have you got a crystal ball over there?

T: Why? What do you see?

P: Well, have you?

T: No, there's no crystal ball there.

P: No, I mean, well, it seems all wrapped up with that same dog.

T: Which dog is that?

P: My dog.

T: Oh, Rover? What's he doing?

P: Just sitting there, and I hope he stays there too.

T: Really?

P: Yes. Now that's funny, isn't it? I know he isn't there and yet I see him.

T: What do you mean, you know he isn't there?

P: I know it's impossible.

T: Doesn't he look real to you?
P: Well, sort of.
T: Well, he looks like a regular dog, doesn't he?
P: Sort of.
T: What's he doing?
P: Just sitting there looking at me.
T: How does he look?
P: [Laughs.] As if I have done him an injustice, I think.
T: You want him to stay over there?
P: Yes!
T: You don't think you can make up with him after all these years?
P: Well, I am not sure.
T: Do you think you can make any gesture of friendship to him?
P: Well, I can feel sorry for him, is that a gesture of friendship?
T: In part. Why don't you call him over?
P: Well, he might come running and I wouldn't like that.
T: Why don't you try and see? Do you have enough courage?
P: Oh, I think I have enough courage.
T: Why don't you make friends with him? Try!
P: If he really were there I think I could, I really do.
T: Well, you see him, don't you?
P: But only in my mind's eye. But I really think I could if he were really there.
T: Why do you say only in your mind's eye? How real does he appear?
P: He looks very real. I mean, like the memories this morning looked.
T: Try calling him over to you.

P: But he isn't there. If he really were . . .

T: Try it and see what he does.

P: All right. Rover, come over, come over slowly. In my mind's eye he is walking over slowly.

T: Forget about this "mind's eye." He's right out there.

P: But he isn't really.

T: You don't want him to be there, do you?

P: No, I kind of think I do.

T: All right.

P: I kinda think I do. I think, I could, yes, I wish he were there.

T: All right, let him be then.

P: Yes, I think he is there.

T: All right. What do you want to do?

P: I think I would like him to come over.

T: Ask him.

P: All right, Rover, come on over. And he does.

T: Where is he?

P: He is on my lap and I am not afraid.

T: He's on your lap?

P: And I'm not afraid.

T: Can you stroke and pet him?

P: Yes.

T: Let me see you.

P: [Stroking.] I am not afraid. I really wish he were actually there.

T: You still won't let yourself believe he is there.

P: Is that it? No, I mean really, so that I could touch him with my hands. I think I would not have that repulsion of touching him with my hands. I think I wouldn't.

T: Why do you think that you won't let yourself if he's sitting there on your lap? Are you trying to make plain that this is just imagination?

P: No, I don't think so. No, I don't think so.

T: Because this morning, if you remember, you went to the dentist.

P: Yes.

T: Certainly there was real physical pain and yet you were able to control that.

P: Yes.

T: Is it so much more impossible to have the little dog here with you?

P: No, I guess not really.

T: Not if you *really* want him.

P: Uh-huh.

T: Where is the dog?

P: He is still on my lap.

T: Let's see.

P: He's still right here.

T: Where is his head?

P: His head's on my lap.

T: What's he doing?

P: He's just lying there.

T: Is he friendly?

P: Yes, and he feels sort of quivery underneath but I don't mind it.

T: Would you like to take him home with you?

P: Well, let's say Judy would like it; yes, I think I would, I would.

T: You don't have to, of course, unless you want to.

P: Well, now, what would you do with a dog in your office?

T: That's a good question. [Patient and therapist laugh together.] I'd have to walk him.

P: You surely would, wouldn't you? Well, maybe you have another patient that could use him.

T: Well, would you like him?

P: [With increasing resolution] Yes, I think I'll take this dog. Yes, I think so!

T: I think under the circumstances if you do that, it might be a good idea to sort of keep this between you and I.

P: [Laughs.] Yes, I think so or they'll commit both of us. Well, no, but really and yet in my memory I could see that dog as plainly as I could see those incidents in my life this morning.

T: How real is he in there sitting on your lap?

P: I think I feel very real, I think so, doctor. I think so.

T: Why don't you take this dog along with you? And as I said, we will keep it a secret between you and I for obvious reasons. Other people wouldn't be able to see or understand this dog anyway. But you'll find in the next day or two, until we meet again and at odd moments, especially at night and the like, that he will be there with you and you will be able to see him very clearly, very vividly. Other people, of course, won't be able to, but you will, and you will be able to make friends with him if you want to.

P: Sort of like Harvey's rabbit, isn't it?

T: A little bit. And of course, you can say that Harvey's rabbit was a figment of imagination but, on the other hand, he was very real to Harvey.

P: Uh-huh. It was real to Harvey, wasn't it?

T: Now, why don't you go back to sleep for me and I will tell you some of this again. [Hypnosis is induced.] I'm going to give you this little dog, Rover, to take with you, this little black dog of your girlhood days. You can take him with you and keep him until the next day or two, until we meet again. When you come back next time, I want you to bring him back with you. Now only you and I will know that you've got this dog. I don't want you to tell anyone else. I think perhaps even your husband at this stage might not understand about this little dog and how real he is to you and what he means to you.

But in the next day or two, whenever you're by yourself, especially at night, alone, the little dog will be there. He won't bother you during the day and he won't make a nuisance of himself and he won't inconvenience you by popping up at the wrong time, none of these things. He's gotten pretty well trained over the years. But there will be little Rover there when you want him to be, when you want to renew your acquaintance with him, when you want to become friends with him. So that this is a way of going back, of going back and undoing the past, giving you a chance to set right the things that went wrong when you were a little girl. To make up with this little dog that you couldn't help, of course, but blame under the circumstances. It's a chance now, as an adult, to really become acquainted with Rover and what he was really like. Not as you saw and thought about him as a little girl, but how he really was.

So this will be a little dog, your little dog, little Rover, the same dog that you had as a little girl. In the next few days, if you can let yourself, I want you to become very well acquainted with him, very well acquainted with him. So that you can see Rover as he really was and really is, rather than the way you saw him as a little girl, rather than the way you remembered him. This will really be Rover, friendly little Rover. Sleep deep. Sleep well. When you awaken, I want you to awaken as if from a deep sleep. You will have no real conscious memory of the suggestion that I have given you here. You will not try to remember, you will not want to remember what I've told you here. But, nevertheless, you will find if you want to make friends with Rover, if you really want it, that he will be with you the next couple of days, he will be with you the next couple of days. If you really want to make friends with him you will be able to. You will be able to get to know this little dog, the dog which held so much terror for you through the years unconsciously. The little dog, you can hardly say, I don't think, that it is a figment of your imagination because actually he has been very real in his consequences. Certainly your feelings about him have been very real. He will be just as real to you as your feelings have been about him. Remember, it is a secret between us. You will have complete control of him. He won't pop up at inconvenient times. Instead, when it is convenient for you, you will be able to renew your association with him.

Now I think we have covered an awful lot of territory in a short period of time. I think perhaps the next session should be our last for a while. I want you to mull it over and think about it, and if you find the decision agreeable, to come to it independently. As I said before, I don't think you are going to be able to be completely cured of this just overnight. It has existed too long and gone too deeply, but I do believe sincerely that you will gradually get used to dogs again. And especially if you are able to make friends with little Rover. So you think it over and in the time between now and the next session, the pieces of our jigsaw puzzle will continue to fall in place.

At your own pace of course, you will be able to face up to much of the past and integrate it and understand and organize it and always the central theme of how the dog fits into this. So that, as I said, when you come the next session, I want you to have thought over whether it will be a convenient point in which to stop for a little while — perhaps for a month and then have another session. You think it over and next session or perhaps the session after that — only one or two more sessions, I believe, should see us well advanced towards a solution of your problem. [The patient is awakened.]

It certainly gets bright, doesn't it [alluding to the sunlight through the window]?

P: Doesn't it?

T: Well, how do you feel? Real good?

P: Fine, fine! Preston is getting real curious about the tape.

T: Is he? Why don't you tell him that it is always available?

P: Well, I don't want him to hear it until it's finished. I think that's better, don't you? It's sort of like starting to read something and then have to wait until the magazine comes next month to finish it. He isn't impatient; he's just curious and anxious. There must be an awful lot of tape, it must take a long time to listen to.

T: Well, I imagine we have about eight or nine hours of tape now.

P: Really? Gosh, he'll have to take a day off for that, won't he?

T: It's nothing that he will be able to do in an evening.

P: No, I think he was aware of that, but I wasn't. He has a more orderly mind, I guess. Well, when one listens to it, it'll have to be sessions then, he can't listen to it all at once. I think he would grow weary listening to it. I want to listen to it with him, may I?

T: Sure.